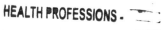
HEALTH PROFESSIONS .

TABLE OF CONTENTS

Secret Key #1 – Time is Your Greatest Enemy

To succeed, you must ration your time properly. The reason that time is so critical is that every question counts the same toward your final score. If you run out of time on any section, the questions that you do not answer will hurt your score far more than earlier questions that you spent extra time on and feel certain are correct.

Success Strategy #1

Pace Yourself

Wear a watch to the PSB H.O. exam. At the beginning of the test, check the time (or start a chronometer on your watch to count the minutes), and check the time after each passage or every few questions to make sure you are "on schedule."

If you find that you are falling behind time during the test, you must speed up. Even though a rushed answer is more likely to be incorrect, it is better to miss a couple of questions by being rushed, than to completely miss later questions by not having enough time. It is better to end with more time than you need than to run out of time.

If you are forced to speed up, do it efficiently. Usually one or more answer choices can be eliminated without too much difficulty. Above all, don't panic. Don't speed up and just begin guessing at random choices. By pacing yourself, and continually monitoring your progress against your watch, you will always know exactly how far ahead or behind you are with your available time. If you find that you are a few minutes behind on a section, don't skip questions without spending any time on it, just to catch back up. Begin spending a little less time per question and after a few questions, you will have caught back up more gradually. Once you catch back up, you can continue working each problem at your normal pace. If you have time at the end, go back then and finish the questions that you left behind.

Furthermore, don't dwell on the problems that you were rushed on. If a problem was taking up too much time and you made a hurried guess, it must have been difficult. The difficult questions are the ones you are most likely to miss anyway, so it isn't a big loss. If you have time left over, as you review the skipped questions, start at the earliest skipped question, spend at most another minute, and then move on to the next skipped question.

Always mark skipped questions in your workbook, NOT on the Scantron. Last minute guessing will be covered in the next chapter.

Lastly, sometimes it is beneficial to slow down if you are constantly getting ahead of time. You are always more likely to catch a careless mistake by working more slowly than quickly, and among very high-scoring students (those who are likely to have lots of time left over), careless errors affect the score more than mastery of material.

Scanning
Don't waste time reading, enjoying, and completely understanding the passage. Simply scan the passage to get a rough idea of what it is about. You will return to the passage for each question, so there is no need to memorize it. Only spend as much time scanning as is necessary to get a vague impression of its overall subject content.

Secret Key #2 – Guessing is not guesswork.

Most students do not understand the impact that proper guessing can have on their score. Unless you score extremely high, guessing will contribute a significant amount of points to your score.

Monkeys Take the PSB H.O. Exam

What most students don't realize is that to insure that random 25% chance, you have to guess randomly. If you put 20 monkeys in a room to take the PSB H.O. exam, assuming they answered once per question and behaved themselves, on average they would get 25% of the questions correct. Put 20 students in the room, and the average will be much lower among guessed questions. Why?

1. The PSB H.O. exam intentionally has deceptive answer choices that "look" right. A student has no idea about a question, so picks the "best looking" answer, which is often wrong. The monkey has no idea what looks good and what doesn't, so will consistently be lucky about 25% of the time.
2. Students will eliminate answer choices from the guessing pool based on a hunch or intuition. Simple but correct answers often get excluded, leaving a 0% chance of being correct. The monkey has no clue, and often gets lucky with the best choice.

This is why the process of elimination endorsed by most test courses is flawed and detrimental to your performance- students don't guess, they make an ignorant stab in the dark that is usually worse than random.

Success Strategy #2

Let me introduce one of the most valuable ideas of this course- the $5 challenge:

You only mark your "best guess" if you are willing to bet $5 on it.
You only eliminate choices from guessing if you are willing to bet $5 on it.

Why $5? Five dollars is an amount of money that is small yet not insignificant, and can really add up fast (20 questions could cost you $100). Likewise, each answer choice on one question of the PSB H.O. exam will have a small impact on your overall score, but it can really add up to a lot of points in the end.

The process of elimination IS valuable. The following shows your chance of guessing it right:

If you eliminate this many choices:	0	1	2	3
Chance of getting it correct	25%	33%	50%	100%

However, if you accidentally eliminate the right answer or go on a hunch for an incorrect answer, your chances drop dramatically: to 0%. By guessing among all the answer choices, you are GUARANTEED to have a shot at the right answer.

- 10 -

That's why the $5 test is so valuable- if you give up the advantage and safety of a pure guess, it had better be worth the risk.

What we still haven't covered is how to be sure that whatever guess you make is truly random. Here's the easiest way:

Always pick the first answer choice among those remaining.

Such a technique means that you have decided, **before you see a single test question**, exactly how you are going to guess- and since the order of choices tells you nothing about which one is correct, this guessing technique is perfectly random.

Specific Guessing Techniques

Similar Answer Choices
When you have two answer choices that are direct opposites, one of them is usually the correct answer.
Example:
A.) forward
B.) backward

These two answer choices are very similar and fall into the same family of answer choices. A family of answer choices is when two or three answer choices are very similar. Often two will be opposites and one may show an equality.
Example:
A.) excited
B.) overjoyed
C.) thrilled
D.) upset

Note how the first three choices are all related. They all ask describe a state of happiness. However, choice D is not in the same family of questions. Being upset is the direct opposite of happiness.

Summary of Guessing Techniques
1. Eliminate as many choices as you can by using the $5 test. Use the common guessing strategies to help in the elimination process, but only eliminate choices that pass the $5 test.
2. Among the remaining choices, only pick your "best guess" if it passes the $5 test.
3. Otherwise, guess randomly by picking the first remaining choice that was not eliminated.

Secret Key #3 – Practice Smarter, Not Harder

Many students delay the test preparation process because they dread the awful amounts of practice time they think necessary to succeed on the test. We have refined an effective method that will take you only a fraction of the time.

There are a number of "obstacles" in your way on the PSB H.O. exam. Among these are answering questions, finishing in time, and mastering test-taking strategies. All must be executed on the day of the test at peak performance, or your score will suffer. The PSB H.O. exam is a mental marathon that has a large impact on your future.

Just like a marathon runner, it is important to work your way up to the full challenge. So first you just worry about questions, and then time, and finally strategy:

Success Strategy #3

1. Find a good source for PSB H.O. exam practice tests.
2. If you are willing to make a larger time investment (or if you want to really "learn" the material, a time consuming but ultimately valuable endeavor), consider buying one of the better study guides on the market
3. Take a practice test with no time constraints, with all study helps "open book." Take your time with questions and focus on applying the strategies.
4. Take another test, this time with time constraints, with all study helps "open book."
5. Take a final practice test with no open material and time limits.

If you have time to take more practice tests, just repeat step 5. By gradually exposing yourself to the full rigors of the test environment, you will condition your mind to the stress of test day and maximize your success.

Secret Key #4 – Prepare, Don't Procrastinate

Let me state an obvious fact: if you take the PSB H.O. exam three times, you will get three different scores. This is due to the way you feel on test day, the level of preparedness you have, and, despite PSB H.O. exam's claims to the contrary, some tests WILL be easier for you than others.

Since your acceptance will largely depend on your score, you should maximize your chances of success. In order to maximize the likelihood of success, you've got to prepare in advance. This means taking practice tests and spending time learning the information and test taking strategies you will need to succeed.

Since you have to pay a registration fee each time you take the PSB H.O. exam, don't take it as a "practice" test. Feel free to take sample tests on your own, but when you go to take the PSB H.O. exam, be prepared, be focused, and do your best the first time!

Secret Key #5 – Test Yourself

Everyone knows that time is money. There is no need to spend too much of your time or too little of your time preparing for the PSB H.O. exam. You should only spend as much of your precious time preparing as is necessary for you to pass it.

Once you have taken a practice test under real conditions of time constraints, then you will know if you are ready for the test or not.

If you have scored extremely high the first time that you take the practice test, then there is not much point in spending countless hours studying. You are already there.

Benchmark your abilities by retaking practice tests and seeing how much you have improved. Once you score high enough to get accepted into the school of your choice, then you are ready.

If you have scored well below where you need, then knuckle down and begin studying in earnest. Check your improvement regularly through the use of practice tests under real conditions. Above all, don't worry, panic, or give up. The key is perseverance!

Then, when you go to take the PSB H.O. exam, remain confident and remember how well you did on the practice tests. If you can score high enough on a practice test, then you can do the same on the real thing.

Top 20 Test Taking Tips

1. Carefully follow all the test registration procedures
2. Know the test directions, duration, topics, question types, how many questions
3. Setup a flexible study schedule at least 3-4 weeks before test day
4. Study during the time of day you are most alert, relaxed, and stress free
5. Maximize your learning style; visual learner use visual study aids, auditory learner use auditory study aids
6. Focus on your weakest knowledge base
7. Find a study partner to review with and help clarify questions
8. Practice, practice, practice
9. Get a good night's sleep; don't try to cram the night before the test
10. Eat a well balanced meal
11. Know the exact physical location of the testing site; drive the route to the site prior to test day
12. Bring a set of ear plugs; the testing center could be noisy
13. Wear comfortable, loose fitting, layered clothing to the testing center; prepare for it to be either cold or hot during the test
14. Bring at least 2 current forms of ID to the testing center
15. Arrive to the test early; be prepared to wait and be patient
16. Eliminate the obviously wrong answer choices, then guess the first remaining choice
17. Pace yourself; don't rush, but keep working and move on if you get stuck
18. Maintain a positive attitude even if the test is going poorly
19. Keep your first answer unless you are positive it is wrong
20. Check your work, don't make a careless mistake

General Strategies

The most important thing you can do is to ignore your fears and jump into the test immediately- do not be overwhelmed by any strange-sounding terms. You have to jump into the test like jumping into a pool- all at once is the easiest way.

Make Predictions

As you read and understand the question, try to guess what the answer will be. Remember that several of the answer choices are wrong, and once you begin reading them, your mind will immediately become cluttered with answer choices designed to throw you off. Your mind is typically the most focused immediately after you have read the question and digested its contents. If you can, try to predict what the correct answer will be. You may be surprised at what you can predict.

Quickly scan the choices and see if your prediction is in the listed answer choices. If it is, then you can be quite confident that you have the right answer. It still won't hurt to check the other answer choices, but most of the time, you've got it!

Answer the Question

It may seem obvious to only pick answer choices that answer the question, but the test writers can create some excellent answer choices that are wrong. Don't pick an answer just because it sounds right, or you believe it to be true. It MUST answer the question. Once you've made your selection, always go back and check it against the question and make sure that you didn't misread the question, and the answer choice does answer the question posed.

Benchmark

After you read the first answer choice, decide if you think it sounds correct or not. If it doesn't, move on to the next answer choice. If it does, mentally mark that answer choice. This doesn't mean that you've definitely selected it as your answer choice, it just means that it's the best you've seen thus far. Go ahead and read the next choice. If the next choice is worse than the one you've already selected, keep going to the next answer choice. If the next choice is better than the choice you've already selected, mentally mark the new answer choice as your best guess.

The first answer choice that you select becomes your standard. Every other answer choice must be benchmarked against that standard. That choice is correct until proven otherwise by another answer choice beating it out. Once you've decided that no other answer choice seems as good, do one final check to ensure that your answer choice answers the question posed.

Valid Information

Don't discount any of the information provided in the question. Every piece of information may be necessary to determine the correct answer. None of the information in the question is there to throw you off (while the answer choices will certainly have information to throw you off). If two seemingly unrelated topics are discussed, don't ignore either. You can be confident there is a relationship, or it wouldn't be included in the question, and you are probably going to have to determine what is that relationship to find the answer.

Avoid "Fact Traps"

Don't get distracted by a choice that is factually true. Your search is for the answer that answers the question. Stay focused and don't fall for an answer that is true but incorrect. Always go back to the question and make sure you're choosing an answer that actually answers the question and is not just a true statement. An answer can be factually correct, but it MUST answer the question asked. Additionally, two answers can both be seemingly correct, so be sure to read all of the answer choices, and make sure that you get the one that BEST answers the question.

Milk the Question

Some of the questions may throw you completely off. They might deal with a subject you have not been exposed to, or one that you haven't reviewed in years. While your lack of knowledge about the subject will be a hindrance, the question itself can give you many clues that will help you find the correct answer. Read the question carefully and look for clues. Watch particularly for adjectives and nouns describing difficult terms or words that you don't recognize. Regardless of if you completely understand a word or not, replacing it with a synonym either provided or one you more familiar with may help you to understand what the questions are asking. Rather than wracking your mind about specific detailed information concerning a difficult term or word, try to use mental substitutes that are easier to understand.

The Trap of Familiarity

Don't just choose a word because you recognize it. On difficult questions, you may not recognize a number of words in the answer choices. The test writers don't put "make-believe" words on the test; so don't think that just because you only recognize all the words in one answer choice means that answer choice must be correct. If you only recognize words in one answer choice, then focus on that one. Is it correct? Try your best to determine if it is correct. If it is, that is great, but if it doesn't, eliminate it. Each word and answer choice you eliminate increases your chances of getting the question correct, even if you then have to guess among the unfamiliar choices.

Eliminate Answers

Eliminate choices as soon as you realize they are wrong. But be careful! Make sure you consider all of the possible answer choices. Just because one appears right, doesn't mean that the next one won't be even better! The test writers will usually put more than one good answer choice for every question, so read all of them. Don't worry if you are stuck between two that seem right. By getting down to just two

- 18 -

remaining possible choices, your odds are now 50/50. Rather than wasting too much time, play the odds. You are guessing, but guessing wisely, because you've been able to knock out some of the answer choices that you know are wrong. If you are eliminating choices and realize that the last answer choice you are left with is also obviously wrong, don't panic. Start over and consider each choice again. There may easily be something that you missed the first time and will realize on the second pass.

Tough Questions
If you are stumped on a problem or it appears too hard or too difficult, don't waste time. Move on! Remember though, if you can quickly check for obviously incorrect answer choices, your chances of guessing correctly are greatly improved. Before you completely give up, at least try to knock out a couple of possible answers. Eliminate what you can and then guess at the remaining answer choices before moving on.

Brainstorm
If you get stuck on a difficult question, spend a few seconds quickly brainstorming. Run through the complete list of possible answer choices. Look at each choice and ask yourself, "Could this answer the question satisfactorily?" Go through each answer choice and consider it independently of the other. By systematically going through all possibilities, you may find something that you would otherwise overlook. Remember that when you get stuck, it's important to try to keep moving.

Read Carefully
Understand the problem. Read the question and answer choices carefully. Don't miss the question because you misread the terms. You have plenty of time to read each question thoroughly and make sure you understand what is being asked. Yet a happy medium must be attained, so don't waste too much time. You must read carefully, but efficiently.

Face Value
When in doubt, use common sense. Always accept the situation in the problem at face value. Don't read too much into it. These problems will not require you to make huge leaps of logic. The test writers aren't trying to throw you off with a cheap trick. If you have to go beyond creativity and make a leap of logic in order to have an answer choice answer the question, then you should look at the other answer choices. Don't overcomplicate the problem by creating theoretical relationships or explanations that will warp time or space. These are normal problems rooted in reality. It's just that the applicable relationship or explanation may not be readily apparent and you have to figure things out. Use your common sense to interpret anything that isn't clear.

Prefixes
If you're having trouble with a word in the question or answer choices, try

dissecting it. Take advantage of every clue that the word might include. Prefixes and suffixes can be a huge help. Usually they allow you to determine a basic meaning. Pre- means before, post- means after, pro - is positive, de- is negative. From these prefixes and suffixes, you can get an idea of the general meaning of the word and try to put it into context. Beware though of any traps. Just because con is the opposite of pro, doesn't necessarily mean congress is the opposite of progress!

Hedge Phrases
Watch out for critical "hedge" phrases, such as likely, may, can, will often, sometimes, often, almost, mostly, usually, generally, rarely, sometimes. Question writers insert these hedge phrases to cover every possibility. Often an answer choice will be wrong simply because it leaves no room for exception. Avoid answer choices that have definitive words like "exactly," and "always".

Switchback Words
Stay alert for "switchbacks". These are the words and phrases frequently used to alert you to shifts in thought. The most common switchback word is "but". Others include although, however, nevertheless, on the other hand, even though, while, in spite of, despite, regardless of.

New Information
Correct answer choices will rarely have completely new information included. Answer choices typically are straightforward reflections of the material asked about and will directly relate to the question. If a new piece of information is included in an answer choice that doesn't even seem to relate to the topic being asked about, then that answer choice is likely incorrect. All of the information needed to answer the question is usually provided for you, and so you should not have to make guesses that are unsupported or choose answer choices that require unknown information that cannot be reasoned on its own.

Time Management
On technical questions, don't get lost on the technical terms. Don't spend too much time on any one question. If you don't know what a term means, then since you don't have a dictionary, odds are you aren't going to get much further. You should immediately recognize terms as whether or not you know them. If you don't, work with the other clues that you have, the other answer choices and terms provided, but don't waste too much time trying to figure out a difficult term.

Contextual Clues
Look for contextual clues. An answer can be right but not correct. The contextual clues will help you find the answer that is most right and is correct. Understand the context in which a phrase or statement is made. This will help you make important distinctions.

Don't Panic

Panicking will not answer any questions for you. Therefore, it isn't helpful. When you first see the question, if your mind goes blank, take a deep breath. Force yourself to mechanically go through the steps of solving the problem and using the strategies you've learned.

Pace Yourself

Don't get clock fever. It's easy to be overwhelmed when you're looking at a page full of questions, your mind is full of random thoughts and feeling confused, and the clock is ticking down faster than you would like. Calm down and maintain the pace that you have set for yourself. As long as you are on track by monitoring your pace, you are guaranteed to have enough time for yourself. When you get to the last few minutes of the test, it may seem like you won't have enough time left, but if you only have as many questions as you should have left at that point, then you're right on track!

Answer Selection

The best way to pick an answer choice is to eliminate all of those that are wrong, until only one is left and confirm that is the correct answer. Sometimes though, an answer choice may immediately look right. Be careful! Take a second to make sure that the other choices are not equally obvious. Don't make a hasty mistake. There are only two times that you should stop before checking other answers. First is when you are positive that the answer choice you have selected is correct. Second is when time is almost out and you have to make a quick guess!

Check Your Work

Since you will probably not know every term listed and the answer to every question, it is important that you get credit for the ones that you do know. Don't miss any questions through careless mistakes. If at all possible, try to take a second to look back over your answer selection and make sure you've selected the correct answer choice and haven't made a costly careless mistake (such as marking an answer choice that you didn't mean to mark). This quick double check should more than pay for itself in caught mistakes for the time it costs.

Beware of Directly Quoted Answers

Sometimes an answer choice will repeat word for word a portion of the question or reference section. However, beware of such exact duplication – it may be a trap! More than likely, the correct choice will paraphrase or summarize a point, rather than being exactly the same wording.

Slang

Scientific sounding answers are better than slang ones. An answer choice that begins "To compare the outcomes..." is much more likely to be correct than one that begins "Because some people insisted..."

Extreme Statements

Avoid wild answers that throw out highly controversial ideas that are proclaimed as established fact. An answer choice that states the "process should used in certain situations, if…" is much more likely to be correct than one that states the "process should be discontinued completely." The first is a calm rational statement and doesn't even make a definitive, uncompromising stance, using a hedge word "if" to provide wiggle room, whereas the second choice is a radical idea and far more extreme.

Answer Choice Families

When you have two or more answer choices that are direct opposites or parallels, one of them is usually the correct answer. For instance, if one answer choice states "x increases" and another answer choice states "x decreases" or "y increases," then those two or three answer choices are very similar in construction and fall into the same family of answer choices. A family of answer choices is when two or three answer choices are very similar in construction, and yet often have a directly opposite meaning. Usually the correct answer choice will be in that family of answer choices. The "odd man out" or answer choice that doesn't seem to fit the parallel construction of the other answer choices is more likely to be incorrect.

Exam Overview

Part I (Vocabulary, Arithmetic, and Form Relationships)	(Vocabulary, Arithmetic, and Form Relationships) 30 questions per mini-test
Part II	Spelling Test
Part III	Reading Comprehension
Part IV	Natural Sciences (Chemistry, Biology, Health etc..)
Part V	Vocational Adjustment Index

Part I- Vocabulary Review

The Vocabulary test on the PSB H.O. Exam consists of a total of 30 questions about Word Knowledge.

Word Knowledge

Nearly and Perfect Synonyms

You must determine which of four provided choices has the best similar definition as a certain word. Nearly similar may often be more correct, because the goal is to test your understanding of the nuances, or little differences, between words. A perfect match may not exist, so don't be concerned if your answer choice is not a complete synonym. Focus upon edging closer to the word. Eliminate the words that you know aren't correct first. Then narrow your search. Cross out the words that are the least similar to the main word until you are left with the one that is the most similar.

Prefixes

Take advantage of every clue that the word might include. Prefixes and suffixes can be a huge help. Usually they allow you to determine a basic meaning. Pre- means before, post- means after, pro – is positive, de- is negative. From these prefixes and suffixes, you can get an idea of the general meaning of the word and look for its opposite. Beware though of any traps. Just because con is the opposite of pro, doesn't necessarily mean congress is the opposite of progress! A list of the most common prefixes and suffixes is included in a special report at the end.

Positive vs. Negative

Many words can be easily determined to be a positive word or a negative word. Words such as despicable, gruesome, and bleak are all negative. Words such as ecstatic, praiseworthy, and magnificent are all positive. You will be surprised at how many words can be considered as either positive or negative. Once that is determined, you can quickly eliminate any other words with an opposite meaning and focus on those that have the other characteristic, whether positive or negative.

Word Strength

Part of the challenge is determining the most nearly similar word. This is particularly true when two words seem to be similar. When analyzing a word, determine how strong it is. For example, stupendous and good are both positive words. However, stupendous is a much stronger positive adjective than good. Also, towering or gigantic are stronger words than tall or large. Search for an answer choice that is similar and also has the same strength. If the main word is weak, look for similar words that are also weak. If the main word is strong, look for similar words that are also strong.

Type and Topic

Another key is what type of word is the main word. If the main word is an adjective describing height, then look for the answer to be an adjective describing height as well. Match both the type and topic of the main word. The type refers the parts of speech, whether the word is an adjective, adverb, or verb. The topic refers to what the definition of the word includes, such as sizes or fashion styles.

Form a Sentence

Many words seem more natural in a sentence. *Specious* reasoning, *irresistible* force, and *uncanny* resemblance are just a few of the word combinations that usually go together. When faced with an uncommon word that you barely understand (and on the PSB H.O. exam there will be many), try to put the word in a sentence that makes sense. It will help you to understand the word's meaning and make it easier to determine its opposite. Once you have a good descriptive sentence that utilizes the main word properly, plug in the answer choices and see if the sentence still has the same meaning with each answer choice. The answer choice that maintains the meaning of the sentence is correct!

Use Replacements

Using a sentence is a great help because it puts the word into a proper perspective. Since the PSB H.O. exam actually gives you a sentence, sometimes you don't always have to create your own (though in many cases the sentence won't be helpful). Read the provided sentence, picking out the main word. Then read the sentence again and again, each time replacing the main word with one of the answer choices. The correct answer should "sound" right and fit.
Example: The desert landscape was desolate. Desolate means

    A. cheerful
    B. creepy
    C. excited
    D. forlorn

After reading the example sentence, begin replacing "desolate" with each of the answer choices. Does "the desert landscape was cheerful, creepy, excited, or forlorn" sound right? Deserts are typically hot, empty, and rugged environments, probably not cheerful, or excited. While creepy might sound right, that word would certainly be more appropriate for a haunted house. But "the desert landscape was forlorn" has a certain ring to it and would be correct.

Eliminate Similar Choices

If you don't know the word, don't worry. Look at the answer choices and just use them. Remember that three of the answer choices will always be wrong. If you can find a common relationship between any three answer choices, then you know they are wrong. Find the answer choice that does not have a common relationship to the other answer choices and it will be the correct answer.
Example: Laconic most nearly means
   A. wordy
   B. talkative
   C. expressive
   D. quiet

In this example the first three choices are all similar. Even if you don't know that laconic means the same as quiet, you know that "quiet" must be correct, because the other three choices were all virtually the same. They were all the same, so they must all be wrong. The one that is different must be correct. So, don't worry if you don't know a word. Focus on the answer choices that you do understand and see if you can identify similarities. Even identifying two words that are similar will allow you to eliminate those two answer choices, for they are both wrong, because they are either both right or both wrong (they're similar, remember), so since they can't both be right, they both must be wrong.

Example:
He worked slowly, moving the leather back and forth until it was _____ .
   A. rough
   B. hard
   C. stiff
   D. pliable

In this example the first three choices are all similar and synonyms. Even without knowing what pliable means, it has to be correct, because you know the other three answer choices mean the same thing.

Adjectives Give it Away

Words mean things and are added to the sentence for a reason. Adjectives in particular may be the clue to determining which answer choice is correct.
Example:
The brilliant scientist made several discoveries that were
   A. dull
   B. dazzling

3 5200 00215 8223

Look at the adjectives first to help determine what makes sense. A "brilliant" or smart scientist would make dazzling, rather than dull discoveries. Without that simple adjective, no answer choice is clear.

Use Logic
Ask yourself questions about each answer choice to see if they are logical.
Example:
In the distance, the deep pounding resonance of the drums could be
  A. seen
  B. heard
Would resonating poundings be "seen"? or Would resonating pounding be "heard"?

The Trap of Familiarity
Don't just choose a word because you recognize it. On difficult questions, you may only recognize one or two words. The PSB H.O. exam doesn't put "make-believe words" on the test, so don't think that just because you only recognize one word means that word must be correct. If you don't recognize four words, then focus on the one that you do recognize. Is it correct? Try your best to determine if it fits the sentence. If it does, that is great, but if it doesn't, eliminate it.

Part I- Mathematics Test Review

The Mathematics Test sections of the PSB H.O. exam consists of 30 questions.

-   All numbers used are real numbers.
-   Figures or drawings beside questions are provided as additional information that should be useful in solving the problem. They are drawn fairly accurately, unless the figure is noted as "not drawn to scale".
-   Jagged or straight lines can both be assumed to be straight.
-   Unless otherwise stated, all drawings and figures lie in a plane.

Solving for Variables
Variables are letters that represent an unknown number. You must solve for that unknown number in single variable problems. The main thing to remember is that you can do anything to one side of an equation as long as you do it to the other.

Example: Solve for x in the equation $2x + 3 = 5$.
Answer: First you want to get the "2x" isolated by itself on one side. To do that, first get rid of the 3. Subtract 3 from both sides of the equation $2x + 3 - 3 = 5 - 3$ or $2x = 2$. Now since the x is being multiplied by the 2 in "2x", you must divide by 2 to get rid of it. So, divide both sides by 2, which gives $2x / 2 = 2 / 2$ or $x = 1$.

Drawings

Other problems may describe a geometric shape, such as a triangle or circle, but may not include a drawing of the shape. The PSB H.O. exam is testing whether you can read a description and make appropriate inferences by visualizing the object and related information. There is a simple way to overcome this obstacle. DRAW THE SHAPE! A good drawing (or even a bad drawing) is much easier to understand and interpret than a brief description.

Make a quick drawing or sketch of the shape described. Include any angles or lengths provided in the description. Once you can see the shape, you have already partially solved the problem and will be able to determine the right answer.

Positive/Negative Numbers

Multiplication/Division

A negative multiplied or divided by a negative = a positive number.
Example: $-3 * -4 = 12$; $-6 / -3 = 2$
A negative multiplied by a positive = a negative number.
Example: $-3 * 4 = -12$; $-6 / 3 = -2$

Addition/Subtraction

Treat a negative sign just like a subtraction sign.
Example: $3 + -2 = 3 - 2$ or 1
Remember that you can reverse the numbers while adding or subtracting.
Example: $-4+2 = 2 + -4 = 2 - 4 = -2$
A negative number subtracted from another number is the same as adding a positive number.
Example: $2 - -1 = 2 + 1 = 3$
Beware of making a simple mistake!
Example: An outdoor thermometer drops from $42º$ to $-8º$. By how many degrees has the outside air cooled?
Answer: A common mistake is to say $42º - 8º = 34º$, but that is wrong. It is actually $42º - -8º$ or $42º + 8º = 50º$

Exponents

When exponents are multiplied together, the exponents are added to get the final result.
Example: $x*x = x^2$, where x^1 is implied and $1 + 1 = 2$.
When exponents in parentheses have an exponent, the exponents are multiplied to get the final result.
Example: $(x^3)^2 = x^6$, because $3*2 = 6$.
Another way to think of this is that $(x^3)^2$ is the same as $(x^3)*(x^3)$. Now you can use the multiplication rule given above and add the exponents, $3 + 3 = 6$, so $(x^3)^2 = x^6$

Decimal Exponents (aka Scientific Notation)

This usually involves converting back and forth between scientific notation and decimal numbers (e.g. 0.02 is the same as 2×10^{-2}). There's an old "cheat" to this problem: if the number is less than 1, the number of digits behind the decimal point is the same as the exponent that 10 is raised to in scientific notation, except that the exponent is a negative number; if the number is greater than 1, the exponent of 10 is equal to the number of digits ahead of the decimal point minus 1.

Example: Convert 3000 to decimal notation.

Answer: 3×10^{3}, since 4 digits are ahead of the decimal, the number is greater than 1, and (4-1) = 3.

Example: Convert 0.05 to decimal notation.

Answer: 5×10^{-2}, since the five is two places behind the decimal (remember, the exponent is negative for numbers less than 1).

Any number raised to an exponent of zero is always 1. Also, unless you know what you're doing, always convert scientific notation to "regular" decimal numbers before doing arithmetic, and convert the answer back if necessary to answer the problem.

Area, Volume, and Surface Area

You can count on questions about area, volume, and surface area to be a significant part of the PSB H.O. exam. While commonly used formulas are provided in the actual PSB H.O. exam test book, it is best to become familiar with the formulas beforehand. A list is provided as a special report at the end for your convenience.

Percents

A percent can be converted to a decimal simply by dividing it by 100.

Example: What is 2% of 50?

Answer: 2% = 2/100 or .02, so .02 * 50 = 1

Word Problems

Percents

Example: Ticket sales for this year's annual concert at Minutemaid Park were $125,000. The promoter is predicting that next year's sales, in dollars, will be 40% greater than this year's. How many dollars in ticket sales is the promoter predicting for next year?

Answer: Next year's is 40% greater. 40% = 40/100 = .4, so .4 * $125,000 = $50,000. However, the example stated that next year's would be greater by that amount, so next year's sales would be this year's at $125,000 plus the increase at $50,000.

$125,000 + $50,000 = $175,000

Distances

Example: In a certain triangle, the longest side is 1 foot longer than the second-longest side, and the second-longest side is 1 foot longer than the shortest side. If the perimeter is 30 feet, how many feet long is the shortest side.

Answer: There are three sides, let's call them A, B, and C. A is the longest, B the medium sized, and C the shortest. Because A is described in reference to B's length and B is described in reference to C's length, all calculations should be done off of C, the final reference. Use a variable to represent C's length, "x". This means that C is "x" long, B is "x + 1" because B was 1 foot longer than C, and A is "x + 1 + 1" because A was 1 foot longer than B. To calculate a perimeter you simply add all three sides together, so P = length A + length B + length C, or $(x) + (x + 1) + (x + 1 + 1) = x + x + x + 1 + 1 + 1 = 3x + 3$. You know that the perimeter equals 30 feet, so $3x + 3 = 30$. Subtracting 3 from both sides gives $3x + 3 - 3 = 30 - 3$ or $3x = 27$. Dividing both sides by 3 to get "x" all by itself gives $3x / 3 = 27 / 3$ or $x = 9$. So C = x = 9, and B = x + 1 = 9 + 1 = 10, and A = x + 1 + 1 = 9 + 1 + 1 = 11. A quick check of 9 + 10 + 11 = 30 for the perimeter distance proves that the answer of x = 9 is correct

Ratios

Example: An architect is drawing a scaled blueprint of an apartment building that is to be 100 feet wide and 250 feet long. On the drawing, if the building is 25 inches long, how many inches wide should it be?

Answer: Recognize the word "scaled" to indicate a similar drawing. Similar drawings or shapes can be solved using ratios. First, create the ratio fraction for the missing number, in this case the number of inches wide the drawing should be. The numerator of the first ratio fraction will be the matching known side, in this case "100 feet" wide. The question "100 feet wide is to how many inches wide?" gives us the first fraction of 100 / x. The question "250 feet long is to 25 inches long?" gives us the second fraction of 250 / 25. Again, note that both numerators (100 and 250) are from the same shape. The denominators ("x" and 25) are both from the same shape or drawing as well. Cross multiplication gives 100 * 25 = 250 * x or 2500 = 250x. Dividing both sides by 250 to get x by itself yields 2500 / 250 = 250x / 250 or 10 = x.

Simple Probability

The probability problems on the PSB H.O. exam are fairly straightforward. The basic idea is this: the probability that something will happen is the number of possible ways that something can happen divided by the total number of possible ways for all things that can happen.

Example: I have 20 balloons, 12 are red, 8 are yellow. I give away one yellow balloon; if the next balloon is randomly picked, what is the probability that it will be yellow?

Answer: The probability is 7/19, because after giving one away, there are 7 different ways that the "something" can happen, divided by 19 remaining possibilities.

Ratios

When a question asks about two similar shapes, expect a ratio problem.

Example: The figure below shows 2 triangles, where triangle ABC ~ A'B'C'. In these similar triangles, a = 3, b = 4, c = 5, and a' = 6. What is the value of b'?

Answer: You are given the dimensions of 1 side that is similar on both triangles (a and a'). You are looking for b' and are given the dimensions of b. Therefore you can set up a ratio of a/a' = b/b' or 3/6 = 4/b'. To solve, cross multiply the two sides, multiplying 6*4 = 3*b' or 24 = 3b'. Dividing both sides by 3 (24/3 = 3b'/3) makes 8 = b', so 8 is the answer.

Note many other problems may have opportunities to use a ratio. Look for problems where you are trying to find dimensions for a shape and you have dimensions for a similar shape. These can nearly always be solved by setting up a ratio. Just be careful and set up corresponding measurements in the ratios. First decide what you are being asked for on shape B, represented by a variable, such as x. Then ask yourself, which side on similar shape A is the same size side as x. That is your first ratio fraction, set up a fraction like 2/x if 2 is the similar size side on shape A. Then find a side on each shape that is similar. If 4 is the size of another side on shape A and it corresponds to a side with size 3 on shape B, then your second ratio fraction is 4/3. Note that 2 and 4 are the two numerators in the ratio fractions and are both from shape A. Also note that "x" the unknown side and 3 are both the denominators in the ratio fractions and are both from shape B.

Angles

If you have a two intersecting lines, remember that the sum of all of the angles can only be 360°. In fact, the two angles on either side of each line will add up to 180°. In the example below, on either side of each line, there is a 137° angle and a 43° angle (137° + 43°) = 180°. Also note that opposite angles are equal. For example, the 43° angle is matched by a similar 43° angle on the opposite side of the intersection.

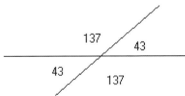

Additionally, parallel lines intersected by a third line will share angles. In the example below, note how each 128° angle is matched by a 128° angle on the opposite side. Also, all of the other angles in this example are 52° angles, because all of the angles on one side of a line have to equal 180° and since there are only two angles, if you have the degree of one, then you can find the degree of the other. In this case, the missing angle is given by 180° − 128° = 52°.

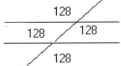

Finally, remember that all of the angles in a triangle will add up to 180°. If you are given two of the angles, then subtract them both from 180° and you will have the degree of the third missing angle.

Example: If you have a triangle with two given angles of 20° and 130°, what degree is the third angle?

Answer: All angles must add up to 180°, so 180° − 20° − 130° = 30°.

Right Triangles

Whenever you see the words "right triangle" or "90° angle," alarm bells should go off. These problems will almost always involve the law of right triangles, AKA The Pythagorean Theorem:

$A^2 + B^2 = C^2$

Where A = the length of one of the shorter sides
B = the length of the other shorter side
C = the length of the hypotenuse or longest side opposite the 90° angle

MAKE SURE YOU KNOW THIS FORMULA. At least 3-5 questions will reference variations on this formula by giving you two of the three variables and asking you to solve for the third.

Example: A right triangle has sides of 3 and 4; what is the length of the hypotenuse?
Answer: Solving the equation, $A^2=9$, $B^2=16$, so $C^2=25$; the square root of 25 is 5, the length of the hypotenuse C.

Example: In the rectangle below, what is the length of the diagonal line?

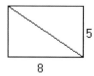

Answer: This rectangle is actually made of two right triangles. Whenever you have a right triangle, the Pythagorean Theorem can be used. Since the right side of the triangle is equal to 5, then the left side must also be equal to 5. This creates a triangle with one side equal to 5 and another side equal to 8. To use the Pythagorean Theorem, we state that $5^2 + 8^2 = C^2$ or $25 + 64 = C^2$ or $89 = C^2$ or C = Square Root of 89

Circles

Many students have never seen the formula for a circle:
$(x-A)^2 + (y-B)^2 = r^2$
This looks intimidating, but it's really not:
A = the coordinate of the center on the x-axis
B = the coordinate of the center on the y-axis
r = the radius of the circle
Example: What is the radius of the circle described by: $(x+2)^2 + (x-3)^2 = 16$
Answer: Since $r^2 = 16$, r, the radius, equals 4.
Also, this circle is centered at (-2,3) since those must be the values of A and B in the generic equation to make it the same as this equation.

Final Note

As mentioned before, word problems describing shapes should always be drawn out. Remember the old adage that a picture is worth a thousand words. If geometric shapes are described (line segments, circles, squares, etc) draw them out rather than trying to visualize how they should look.

Approach problems systematically. Take time to understand what is being asked for. In many cases there is a drawing or graph that you can write on. Draw lines, jot notes, do whatever is necessary to create a visual picture and to allow you to understand what is being asked.

Even if you have always done well in math, you may not succeed on the PSB H.O. exam. While math tests in school will test specific competencies in specific subjects, the PSB H.O. exam frequently tests your ability to apply math concepts from vastly different math subjects in one problem. However, in few cases is any PSB H.O. exam Mathematics Test problem more than two "layers" deep.

What does this mean for you? You can easily learn the PSB H.O. exam Mathematics Test through taking multiple practice tests. If you have some gaps in your math knowledge, we suggest you buy a more basic study guide to help you build a foundation before applying our secrets. Check out our special report to find out which books are worth your time.

Part I – Form Relationship Test

The Part I Form Relationship Test requires you to visualize differences in object and manipulate things mentally.

Rule Busters
Each problem provides you with some known information in the form of angles, odd shapes, shaded sections, etc. These are the rules that you have to work with. Rule busters are answer choices that immediately clash with a rule and can be quickly ruled out.
Example:
An unfolded shaded shape resembles a pyramid shaped object. The base of the pyramid is shaded dark.

This is a rule. Therefore any of the folded shape answer choices that have a base that is light, instead of shaded dark is a rule buster, and is wrong! Quickly scan through the list of answer choices and eliminate all of those that have a light colored pyramid base.

Identify the Odd Shape
Find the most unusual characteristic on the given perspectives and then focus on how that specific perspective would look or fit through the answer choices. Don't waste time on the common features, but find the unusual feature or design and spend your time looking for how it compares to the answer choices.

Process of Elimination
If you can't figure out which one is best, figure out which ones are worst. If you can safely eliminate certain answer choices, then you improve your chances at a guess and with the tight time restrictions you face, guessing will be an important part of your strategy on this particular test section.

Identify the Differences
What is different between the perspectives in the answer choices. Don't waste time looking at the concerns of the perspectives on the answer choices if they all have the same corner design. Focus on the differences and then you can narrow your answer choice down to the correct perspective and answer.

Watch the Dotted Line
A dotted line indicates a wall not clearly seen. Determining when and where the dotted lines should be can quickly eliminate a number of answer choices, as they give you something to hone in on and use as a rule buster. By quickly looking for which answer choices do not have dotted line, on a perspective that you know should have one, then you can usually quickly eliminate a couple of choices.

Draw a Line

The answer choices are all on the same line and also on the same line as one of the given views of the object. Mentally draw a straight horizontal line off of the various points on the given view, such that it intersects each of the choices. You will be able to see where the lines on the given view match up and if there is no line, you should understand why.

Example:

You are provided with the end view of an object that has a line (representing an exposed edge facing you) in its middle. The four answer choices are directly to the right of the provided end view. Mentally draw a horizontal line starting at that middle line on the end view and through each of the answer choices. Any answer choices that do not have an edge that falls on that line can be immediately eliminated.

Pick 2 Sides

For questions that have the shaded sides that you must fold up, don't try to visualize the entire shape. Pick two unique sides on the provided foldout and try to identify them in the answer choices. This should allow you to quickly eliminate the wrong answers and narrow your selection down to the correct choice.

Points or Flat Ends

In picking a unique part of the provided perspective and then comparing it to each of the answer choices, it often helps to consider the tips or points on the provided perspective. Many of the shapes that are shown have either pointed or flat ends or sides. This is a quick rule buster characteristic that you can check each of the answer choices for. If the provided perspective has all flat edges and no points, then any answer choices that have a point, instead of a flat edge, can be immediately eliminated.

Remember It's Flat

Sometimes the foldout perspectives that are shown appear to be shown in a folded out state that is not entirely flat. That is an optical illusion. All foldouts are completely flat, which means that when folded, not all sides will be perpendicular to the others, but will be at a more sloped angle. Don't be fooled. These can be among the easiest problems, because in order to create the optical illusion of 3 dimensions, a completely flat foldout must have certain characteristics that can be easy to check for.

Stop and Look for Similarities

For questions involving cubes with painted sides, once you identify one cube that answers the question, stop and ask yourself what made that cube fit the description. Then methodically go through the stack of cubes and see if any other cubes are in similar locations and would therefore also answer the question or fit the description.

Example:

How many cubes have one of their exposed sides painted?

You realize that one of the cubes on the front row of a towering cube complex has only one side exposed (other than the bottom) which would make that side painted. Understanding that for the cube to only have a single side exposed it must have at least one cube on either side, on top, and behind it. Ask yourself if any other cubes are in that similar situation – DON'T just look around and go through the same process of trying to decipher each cube again. You've already determined the criteria for having a single side painted. Therefore, restrict your search to other cubes that are in a similar setting – perhaps a cube on the back row would also have a cube on either side, on top of, and in this case in front of it.

Use Your Fingers

Unfortunately, on the PSB H.O. exam you won't be provided with a protractor to measure the angles for the questions in which you must rank the angles by size from smallest to largest. However, while you aren't allowed to bring a protractor, you can still use the natural tools that you have in your possession – your fingers. Use your fingers as scissors and hold them up to the first angle and take a "snapshot" of the angle by locking your fingers into the position representing that angle. Then, compare that angle to each of the others in order to determine if they are larger or smaller. Your fingers can be a great tool to use for these problems and can allow you to quickly compare a series of angles and determine the relative size of each.

Make Measurements

If all the lines on the angles shown were the same length, then the problems would be much easier. You would be able to take your pencil and measure the distances between the ends of the lines and whichever angle had the greatest distance would of course be the largest angle. The problem is that the lines are all different lengths, making it nearly impossible to use this method.

However, what if you could make the lines all the same length, then the method would become viable. Fortunately, there are a number of quick methods to making all the lines the same length for this purpose. They all involve using something of consistent width or length as a gauge. For instance, if you had a small piece of paper, the width of a gum wrapper, then you could hold it up to the first angle, such that it nearly hid the vortex of the angle. Then, you could make a quick pencil mark on the paper corresponding to the exposed lines coming out from underneath the piece of paper. If you have the paper held at the correct angle corresponding to the angle of the answer choice, then the marks that you make would represent points that are equidistant from the vortex. By doing this to each of the answer choices, you can make all of the lines on the angles the same length by making these equidistant marks on the paper. Then by going back and comparing the distances between the marks, you can create a gauge of how wide each angle is at that point. The wider the distance between the marks, the larger the angle.

Be careful though. Whenever you perform this type of measurement, it is crucial that you be consistent. The angle you hold the piece of paper at as you make the marks (relative to the angle of the answer choice) MUST be the same as you go from answer choice to answer choice. Also, you must use the same section of the piece of paper each time, to ensure that you eliminate any variance in the width of the piece of paper.

Alternatively, you can also take some given distance, for example the width of the metal part of a common pencil. Hold that section of the pencil up to the angle and slide it up and down the angle until you reach the point at which the ends of the metal piece line up with the width of the angle. By using another pencil as a gauge, you can determine how far down the angle you have to go in order to reach the point that the opening is as wide as the metal piece is long.

By doing this to each of the answer choices, you can then compare distances to that common point (which is the point on the angle that is as wide as the metal part of the pencil). The longer the distance, the more narrow or smaller the angle.

Majority Rules

If you are completely stumped between two angles, and can't determine which is larger, use the answer choices to ease your selection. If three of the answer choices have angle 1 listed as being larger than angle 2, then odds are that angle 1 is larger, so go with the majority in those cases. This should only be used when you are really pressed for time or are completely baffled by one of the problems.

Know When to Move On

Whenever you have identified the angle that you know is the largest, quickly look at your answer choices and determine if there are more than one that have that selection as the largest. If you know that the first angle is the largest, then look for the answer choices that have angle 1 listed last, since the question is asking you to rank the angles from smallest to largest. If only one answer choice has angle 1 listed, last, then you know it must be correct and can immediately move on.

Use Quick Symbology

When you are marking up the answer choices to indicate whether they are larger or smaller, come up with a method of notation that won't be confusing to you. For example, when you're measuring angles, and you know which one is largest, write an "L" down on your scratch paper to correspond to which angle you have identified as largest (you may need to create a 1, 2, 3, 4 on your scratch paper for this purpose). For the smallest, write an "S". For the middle two sizes, write "ML" or "MS", where ML represents the larger of the two middle sizes and MS represents the smaller of the two middle sizes. If you use numbers to rank, you may start to get confused as numbers are also used to list the different angles in the answer choices.

Eyeball the Middle

Since any scale you use to measure distances is going to be relative (this angle is wider than that one), you make have to make multiple measurements to get the final answer.

Example:

If you are using your locked fingers to make angular measurements, then if the first angle you lock your fingers off of is the largest, then all you really know is that the other three are all smaller.

However, if you can lock your fingers on one of the middle angle sizes, then you know which two are either larger or smaller and which one is larger or smaller, considerably narrowing down the problem and probably giving you enough information to make your answer selection.

Therefore before you begin, if you can quickly "eyeball" which of the angles if probably in the middle and then use that as your baseline for measurements, you might have to make fewer follow up measurements.

Crease Distances

For the hole punch problems, look for the distance the hole is from the crease. If you double the distance between a hole and the crease, then you get the distance apart that two holes will be on a card that is only folded once.

2 to the X

Count the number of times the card is folded and calculate 2 to that power or 2^x where x is the number of times the card is folded.

Example: If the card is folded twice, then you take 2^2 or 4 in order to get the number of holes that would be on the resultant card

Be careful though, since PSB H.O. often has unusual folds, this technique does not always work, but it can be a good sanity check if you understand its limitations.

Center Punches

Holes punched away from the center of the initial paper will usually not have a resultant hole near the center, so long as the card is not folded into less than a single quadrant.

Hole punches near the center will usually still be near the center once the paper is unfolded.

Crossing Creases

Remember that holes can only cross creases. If a paper is folded once, then you can mentally draw a line through the holes that is perpendicular to the crease and all unfolded holes would lie upon this line. This strategy works for multiple folds as well, just remember that if you have creases on two sides, then you would have to mentally draw lines through the shown holes going perpendicularly through first the first crease and then another line going perpendicularly through the second crease.

Tough Questions

If you are stumped on a problem or it appears too hard or too difficult, don't waste time. Move on! Remember though, if you can quickly check for obvious "rule busters" your chances of guessing correctly are greatly improved. Before you completely give up, at least check for the easy rule busters, which should knock out a couple of possible answers. Eliminate what you can and then guess at the remainder before moving on.

Part II – Spelling Test

It is extremely difficult to teach someone how to be a good speller, if you have been a bad speller all your life. Becoming a good speller takes lots of time. That is why we have decided to create a link review for this section of this test. Please use the links listed below to work on your spelling to succeed on the PSB H.O. test.

http://www.sentex.net/~mmcadams/spelling.html

http://www.spelling.hemscott.net/

http://eslus.com/LESSONS/SPELL/SPELL.HTM

http://ccc.commnet.edu/grammar/spelling.htm

http://www.esl-lounge.com/quiz-spelling.shtml

http://owl.english.purdue.edu/handouts/grammar/g_spelhomo.html

Part III - Reading Comprehension

Skimming

Your first task when you begin reading is to answer the question "What is the topic of the selection?" This can best be answered by quickly skimming the passage for the general idea, stopping to read only the first sentence of each paragraph. A paragraph's first sentence is usually the main topic sentence, and it gives you a summary of the content of the paragraph.

Once you've skimmed the passage, stopping to read only the first sentences, you will have a general idea about what it is about, as well as what is the expected topic in each paragraph.

Each question will contain clues as to where to find the answer in the passage. Do not just randomly search through the passage for the correct answer to each question. Search scientifically. Find key word(s) or ideas in the question that are going to either contain or be near the correct answer. These are typically nouns, verbs, numbers, or phrases in the question that will probably be duplicated in the passage. Once you have identified those key word(s) or idea, skim the passage quickly to find where those key word(s) or idea appears. The correct answer choice will be nearby.

Example: What caused Martin to suddenly return to Paris?

The key word is Paris. Skim the passage quickly to find where this word appears. The answer will be close by that word.

However, sometimes key words in the question are not repeated in the passage. In those cases, search for the general idea of the question.

Example: Which of the following was the psychological impact of the author's childhood upon the remainder of his life?

Key words are "childhood" or "psychology". While searching for those words, be alert for other words or phrases that have similar meaning, such as "emotional effect" or "mentally" which could be used in the passage, rather than the exact word "psychology".

Numbers or years can be particularly good key words to skim for, as they stand out from the rest of the text.

Example: Which of the following best describes the influence of Monet's work in the 20th century?

20th contains numbers and will easily stand out from the rest of the text. Use 20th as the key word to skim for in the passage.

Other good key word(s) may be in quotation marks. These identify a word or phrase that is copied directly from the passage. In those cases, the word(s) in quotation marks are exactly duplicated in the passage.

Example: In her college years, what was meant by Margaret's "drive for excellence"?

"Drive for excellence" is a direct quote from the passage and should be easy to find.

Once you've quickly found the correct section of the passage to find the answer, focus upon the answer choices. Sometimes a choice will repeat word for word a portion of the passage near the answer. However, beware of such duplication – it may be a trap! More than likely, the correct choice will paraphrase or summarize the related portion of the passage, rather than being exactly the same wording.

For the answers that you think are correct, read them carefully and make sure that they answer the question. An answer can be factually correct, but it MUST answer the question asked. Additionally, two answers can both be seemingly correct, so be sure to read all of the answer choices, and make sure that you get the one that BEST answers the question.

Some questions will not have a key word.

Example: Which of the following would the author of this passage likely agree with?

In these cases, look for key words in the answer choices. Then skim the passage to find where the answer choice occurs. By skimming to find where to look, you can minimize the time required.

Sometimes it may be difficult to identify a good key word in the question to skim for in the passage. In those cases, look for a key word in one of the answer choices to skim for. Often the answer choices can all be found in the same paragraph, which can quickly narrow your search.

Paragraph Focus
Focus upon the first sentence of each paragraph, which is the most important. The main topic of the paragraph is usually there.

Once you've read the first sentence in the paragraph, you have a general idea about what each paragraph will be about. As you read the questions, try to determine which paragraph will have the answer. Paragraphs have a concise topic. The answer should either obviously be there or obviously not. It will save time if you can jump straight to the paragraph, so try to remember what you learned from the first sentences.
Example: The first paragraph is about poets; the second is about poetry. If a question asks about poetry, where will the answer be? The second paragraph.

The main idea of a passage is typically spread across all or most of its paragraphs. Whereas the main idea of a paragraph may be completely different than the main idea of the very next paragraph, a main idea for a passage affects all of the paragraphs in one form or another.
Example: What is the main idea of the passage?

For each answer choice, try to see how many paragraphs are related. It can help to count how many sentences are affected by each choice, but it is best to see how many paragraphs are affected by the choice. Typically the answer choices will include incorrect choices that are main ideas of individual paragraphs, but not the entire passage. That is why it is crucial to choose ideas that are supported by the most paragraphs possible.

Eliminate Choices
Some choices can quickly be eliminated. "Andy Warhol lived there." Is Andy Warhol even mentioned in the article? If not, quickly eliminate it.

When trying to answer a question such as "the passage indicates all of the following EXCEPT" quickly skim the paragraph searching for references to each choice. If the reference exists, scratch it off as a choice. Similar choices may be crossed off simultaneously if they are close enough.

In choices that ask you to choose "which answer choice does NOT describe?" or "all of the following answer choices are identifiable characteristics, EXCEPT which?" look for answers that are similarly worded. Since only one answer can be correct, if there are two answers that appear to mean the same thing, they must BOTH be incorrect, and can be eliminated.
Example:
A.)   changing values and attitudes
B.)   a large population of mobile or uprooted people

These answer choices are similar; they both describe a fluid culture. Because of their similarity, they can be linked together. Since the answer can have only one choice, they can also be eliminated together.

Contextual Clues
Look for contextual clues. An answer can be right but not correct. The contextual clues will help you find the answer that is most right and is correct. Understand the context in which a phrase is stated.

When asked for the implied meaning of a statement made in the passage, immediately go find the statement and read the context it was made in. Also, look for an answer choice that has a similar phrase to the statement in question.
Example: In the passage, what is implied by the phrase "Churches have become more or less part of the furniture"?

Find an answer choice that is similar or describes the phrase "part of the furniture" as that is the key phrase in the question. "Part of the furniture" is a saying that means something is fixed, immovable, or set in their ways. Those are all similar ways of saying "part of the furniture." As such, the correct answer choice will probably include a similar rewording of the expression.
Example: Why was John described as "morally desperate".

The answer will probably have some sort of definition of morals in it. "Morals" refers to a code of right and wrong behavior, so the correct answer choice will likely have words that mean something like that.

Fact/Opinion
When asked about which statement is a fact or opinion, remember that answer choices that are facts will typically have no ambiguous words. For example, how long is a long time? What defines an ordinary person? These ambiguous words of "long" and "ordinary" should not be in a factual statement. However, if all of the

choices have ambiguous words, go to the context of the passage. Often a factual statement may be set out as a research finding.
Example: "The scientist found that the eye reacts quickly to change in light."

Opinions may be set out in the context of words like thought, believed, understood, or wished.
Example: "He thought the Yankees should win the World Series."

Opposites
Answer choices that are direct opposites are usually correct. The paragraph will often contain established relationships (when this goes up, that goes down). The question may ask you to draw conclusions for this and will give two similar answer choices that are opposites.
Example:
A.) a decrease in housing starts
B.) an increase in housing starts

Make Predictions
As you read and understand the passage and then the question, try to guess what the answer will be. Remember that three of the four answer choices are wrong, and once you being reading them, your mind will immediately become cluttered with answer choices designed to throw you off. Your mind is typically the most focused immediately after you have read the passage and question and digested its contents. If you can, try to predict what the correct answer will be. You may be surprised at what you can predict.

Quickly scan the choices and see if your prediction is in the listed answer choices. If it is, then you can be quite confident that you have the right answer. It still won't hurt to check the other answer choices, but most of the time, you've got it!

Answer the Question
It may seem obvious to only pick answer choices that answer the question, but PSB H.O. exam can create some excellent answer choices that are wrong. Don't pick an answer just because it sounds right, or you believe it to be true. It MUST answer the question. Once you've made your selection, always go back and check it against the question and make sure that you didn't misread the question, and the answer choice does answer the question posed.

Benchmark
After you read the first answer choice, decide if you think it sounds correct or not. If it doesn't, move on to the next answer choice. If it does, make a mental note (or rest your pencil tip on the Scantron circle for choice A) about that choice. This doesn't mean that you've definitely selected it as your answer choice, it just means that it's the best you've seen thus far. Go ahead and read the next choice. If the next choice

is worse than the one you've already selected, keep going to the next answer choice. If the next choice is better than the choice you've already selected, then make a mental note about that answer choice.

As you read through the list, you are mentally noting the choice you think is right. That is your new standard. Every other answer choice must be benchmarked against that standard. That choice is correct until proven otherwise by another answer choice beating it out. Once you've decided that no other answer choice seems as good, do one final check to ensure that it answers the question posed.

New Information
Correct answers will usually contain the information listed in the paragraph and question. Rarely will completely new information be inserted into a correct answer choice. Occasionally the new information may be related in a manner than PSB H.O. exam is asking for you to interpret, but seldom.
Example:
The argument above is dependent upon which of the following assumptions?
A.) Charles's Law was used

If Charles's Law is not mentioned at all in the referenced paragraph and argument, then it is unlikely that this choice is correct. All of the information needed to answer the question is provided for you, and so you should not have to make guesses that are unsupported or choose answer choices that have unknown information that cannot be reasoned.

Valid Information
Don't discount any of the information provided in the passage, particularly shorter ones. Every piece of information may be necessary to determine the correct answer. None of the information in the paragraph is there to throw you off (while the answer choices will certainly have information to throw you off). If two seemingly unrelated topics are discussed, don't ignore either. You can be confident there is a relationship, or it wouldn't be included in the paragraph, and you are probably going to have to determine what is that relationship for the answer.

Time Management
In technical passages, do not get lost on the technical terms. Skip them and move on. You want a general understanding of what is going on, not a mastery of the passage.

When you encounter material in the selection that seems difficult to understand, it often may not be necessary and can be skipped. Only spend time trying to understand it if it is going to be relevant for a question. Understand difficult phrases only as a last resort.

Answer general questions before detail questions. A reader with a good understanding of the whole passage can often answer general questions without rereading a word. Get the easier questions out of the way before tackling the more time consuming ones.

Identify each question by type. Usually the wording of a question will tell you whether you can find the answer by referring directly to the passage or by using your reasoning powers. You alone know which question types you customarily handle with ease and which give you trouble and will require more time. Save the difficult questions for last.

Final Warnings

Word Usage Questions
When asked how a word is used in the passage, don't use your existing knowledge of the word. The question is being asked precisely because there is some strange or unusual usage of the word in the passage. Go to the passage and use contextual clues to determine the answer. Don't simply use the popular definition you already know.

Switchback Words
Stay alert for "switchbacks". These are the words and phrases frequently used to alert you to shifts in thought. The most common switchback word is "but". Others include although, however, nevertheless, on the other hand, even though, while, in spite of, despite, regardless of.

Avoid "Fact Traps"
Once you know which paragraph the answer will be in, focus on that paragraph. However, don't get distracted by a choice that is factually true about the paragraph. Your search is for the answer that answers the question, which may be about a tiny aspect in the paragraph. Stay focused and don't fall for an answer that describes the larger picture of the paragraph. Always go back to the question and make sure you're choosing an answer that actually answers the question and is not just a true statement.

Part IV- Natural Sciences Test Review

These questions will test your knowledge of basic principles and concepts in biology, chemistry, and physics.

While a general knowledge of these subjects is important, a complete mastery of them is NOT necessary to succeed on the Science Test. Don't be intimidated by the questions presented. They do not require highly advanced knowledge, but only the ability to recognize common problem types and apply basic principles and concepts to solving them.

That is our goal, to show you the simple methods to solving these problems, so that while you will not gain a mastery of these subjects from this guide, you will learn the methods necessary to succeed on the PSB H.O. exam.

This test may scare you. It may have been years since you've studied some of the basic concepts covered, and for even the most accomplished and studied student, these terms may be unfamiliar. General test-taking skill will help the most. DO NOT run out of time, move quickly, and use the easy pacing methods we outlined in the test-taking tactics section.

The most important thing you can do is to ignore your fears and jump into the test immediately- do not be overwhelmed by any strange-sounding terms. You have to jump into the test like jumping into a pool- all at once is the easiest way. Managing your time on this test can prove to be extremely difficult, as some of the questions may leave you stumped and countless minutes may waste away while you rack your brain for the answer. To be successful though, you must work efficiently and get through the entire test before running out of time.

General Review

Circulatory System

The cardiovascular system is vital for providing oxygen and nutrients to tissues and removing waste. The heart is divided into four chambers-two atria and two ventricles-that communicate through orifices on each side. The right atrium receives blood from the venous system and then lets blood fall down into the right ventricle. Blood then goes to the lungs for a new supply of oxygen. Then the blood comes back from the lungs and goes to the left atrium. It then falls into the left ventricle and is pumped into the general circulation. The heart is composed of three layers: epicardium, myocardium and an endocardium. Heart sounds are due to the vibrations produced by blood and valve movements. Blood pressure is the force exerted by blood against the insides of the blood vessels. Heart rate is determined by physical activity, body temperature, and concentration of ions. The heart is controlled by impulses from the S-A node which passes to the A-V node.

The arterial system is responsible for delivering oxygen to various tissues and the venous system is responsible for removing waste and returning blood to the heart.

Hypertension, is characterized by elevated arterial pressure and is one of the more common diseases of the cardiovascular system. Arteriosclerosis is accompanied by decreased elasticity of the arterial walls and followed by narrowing of the lumen. Hormones can also play a large role in blood pressure regulation. The hormone *aldosterone* can promote retention of water in the kidneys and increased blood volume, which in turn increases blood pressure.

Key Terms

Tachycardia-abnormally fast heartbeat
Bradycardia-abnormally slow heartbeat
Fibrillation-rapid heart beats
Red blood cell (erythrocyte)- transports carbon dioxide and oxygen
White blood cell (leukocyte)- fight infection including neutrophils, eosinophils, and basophils

Blood is made up of approximately 45% hematocrit, and 55% plasma. Plasma is primarily water, however contains approx. 7% protein and 1.5 other substances. The proteins found in plasma are: albumin, globulin and fibrinogen. Hematocrit is made up of mostly red blood cells, but also white blood cells and platelets. Platelets can be key in blood clotting to form a plug.

Respiratory Review

The respiratory stem includes the nose, nasal cavity, sinuses, pharynx, larynx, trachea, bronchial tree, and lungs. Air enters the nose, travels through the nasal cavity where the air is warmed. The air goes through the pharynx, which functions as a common duct for air and food. Then the larynx, which is at the top of the trachea and holds the vocal cords allows passage of air. The trachea divides into the right and left bronchi on the way into the bronchial tree and the lungs.

The right lung has three lobes and the left lung has two lobes. Gas exchange occurs between the air and the blood within the alveoli, which are tiny air sacs. Diffusion is the mechanism by which oxygen and carbon dioxide are exchanged.

Breathing is controlled by the medulla oblongata and pons. Inspiration is controlled by changes in the thoracic cavity. Air fills the lung because of atmospheric pressure pushing air in. Expansion of the lungs is aided by surface tension, which holds pleural membranes together. In addition, the diaphragm, which is located just below the lungs, and stimulated by phrenic nerve acts as a suction pump to encourage inspiration. Expiration comes from the recoil of tissues and the surface tension of the alveoli.

Aerobic respiration occurs in the presence of oxygen and mostly takes place in the mitochondria of a cell. Anaerobic respiration occurs in the absence of oxygen and takes place in the cytoplasm of a cell. Both of these mechanisms occur in cellular respiration in humans. With anaerobic respiration glucose is broken down and produces less ATP when compared to aerobic respiration.

Key Terms

Anoxia- absence of oxygen in tissue
Atelectasis- collapse of a lung
Dyspnea- difficulty in the breathing cycle
Hypercapnia- excessive carbon dioxide in the blood
Tidal Volume-amount of air that normally moves in and out of the lungs

Nervous System

The nervous system is made of the central nervous system (CNS) and the peripheral nervous system (PNS). The central nervous system is made up of the brain and the spinal cord. The peripheral nervous system consists of cranial and spinal nerves that innervate organs, muscles and sensory systems. The brain controls: thought, reasoning, memory, sight, and judgement. The brain is made up of four lobes: frontal, parietal, temporal, and occipital. The spinal cord is a made up of neural tracts that conduct information to and from the brain.

Cranial nerves in the peripheral nervous system connect the brain to the head, neck and truck. Peripheral nerves allow control of muscle groups in the upper and lower extremities and sensory stimulation. The peripheral nerves are spinal nerves that branch off the spinal cord going toward organs, and muscles.

The autonomic nervous system controls reflexive functions of the brain. Including "fight or flight" response and maintaining homeostasis. Homeostasis is a state of equilibrium within tissues. The autonomic nervous system uses neurotransmitters to help conduct nerve signals and turn on/off various cell groups.

Nervous tissue is composed of neurons, which are the functional unit of the nervous system. A neuron includes a cell body, and organelles usually found in cells. Dendrites provide receptive information to the neuron and a single axon carries the information away.

Synapse- junction between two neurons
Action potential- threshold at which neurons fire

Digestive System

Digestion is a process that food is absorbed. The mouth begins to prepare food for digestion. Teeth grind food into smaller substrates. Then salivary glands, which secrete saliva, begin digestion of the food using enzymes. The pharynx and esophagus allow passage of the food into the stomach. The stomach uses gastric juices and absorbs a small amount of the food. Then, the food goes to the small intestine. The pancreas and the liver release enzymes and bile respectively into the small intestine to aid in absorption. The small intestine is composed of the duodenum, jejunum, and ileum. Then, substrates are passed into the large intestine, which has little digestive function. Absorption of water and electrolytes does occur in the large intestine.

Peristalsis is the wave like movement occurring in the digestive system that propels food downward. The alimentary canal is the path food travels from the mouth to the anus. Feces are composed mostly of water and substrates and are not absorbed.

Key Terms

Colelithiasis- stones in the gallbladder
Diverticulitis- inflammation of the small pouches in the colon, if present
Hepatitis- inflammation of the liver
Somatitis- inflammation of the mouth
Dyspepsia- indigestion
Enteritis- inflammation of the intestine

Reproductive System

Male reproductive organs are specialized for the formation of sperm (gamete) and transporting sperm. The vas deferens is the tube that sperm travels through. Semen is composed of sperm cells and secretions of the prostate and bulbourethral glands. Semen activates sperm cells.

Testosterone is the most important male hormone. Testosterone encourages the development of male sex organs. It is responsible for the development of male secondary sexual characteristics.

Female reproductive organs are specialized for childbirth and development of a fetus. The primary structures are the ovaries, uterus, and vagina. The ovaries release an egg cell (gamete) into the uterus. The uterus sustains life for the embryo until childbirth. The vagina allows transportation of the fetus during delivery.

Estrogen and progesterone are the primary female sex hormones. Estrogen is responsible for female sexual characteristics. Progesterone is responsible for changes in the uterus. Menopause is related to low estrogen levels and changes in the female reproductive organs. The product of fertilization is a zygote with 46 chromosomes.

Key Terms

Amenorrhea- absence of menstrual flow
Gestation- 40 weeks of pregnancy
Orchitis- inflammation of a testis
Cesarean section- birth of a fetus through an abdominal incision

Urinary System

The urinary system consists of the kidneys, ureters, bladder, and urethra. The kidney functions to remove metabolic wastes from the blood and excrete them. They also help regulate blood pressure, pH of the blood, and red blood cell production. The basic functional unit of the kidney is the nephron. The nephron consists of a renal corpuscle and a renal tubule. Urine is the end product of the urinary system. The kidneys are involved in filtration, re-absorption and secretion. Glomerular filtration is regulated by osmotic pressure.

The ureter is a tube that connects the kidneys and the bladder. Kidney stones can become lodged in the ureter. Peristaltic waves in the ureter force urine to the bladder. The bladder stores urine and forces urine into the urethra. Muscle fibers in the wall of the bladder form the detrusor muscle.

Key Terms

Enuresis-uncontrolled urination
Dieuretic- a substance that encourages urination
Pyuria- pus in the urine
Ureteritis- inflammation of the ureter

Ear

The external ear collects sound and passes the sound to the tympanic membrance. Then the middle ear increases the force of the sound waves using the malleus, stapes, and incus. Auditory tubes connect the middle ear to throat and help maintain proper pressure. The inner ear consists of complex system of tubes and chambers-occeous, membranous labyrinths and also the cochlea. Auditory impulses are interpreted in the temporal lobes.

Eye

The wall of the eye has an outer, middle and inner layer. The sclera (outer layer) is protective. The cornea refracts light entering the eye and is found on the anterior aspect of the sclera. The choroid coat (middle layer) helps keep the inside of the eye dark. The retina (inner layer) contains the receptor cells. The visual receptors are rods and cones. Rods are responsible for colorless vision in dim light, and cones are responsible for color vision.

Key Terms

Otitis media- inflammation of the middle ear
Diplopia- double vision
Tinnitus- ringing in the ears
Vertigo-sensation of dizziness

Element Review

Fluorine, Chlorine, Bromide and Iodine are all halogens also known as salt formers. Helium, Neon, Argon, Krypton and Xenon are all inert gases also known as noble gases.
Lithium, Sodium, Potassium, Rubidium, and Cesium are all alkali metals.

The following periodic table presentation of Chlorine can be broken down into the following:

17	-	Atomic number
Cl	-	Element symbol
Chlorine	-	Element name
34.45	-	Atomic Weight

The horizontal rows of the periodic table are called periods. From left to right these are arranged by increasing atomic numbers. The vertical rows have similar chemical similarities. The number of known chemical elements is 109. The periodic table was created by, Dmitri Mendeleev a Russian chemist.

An atom is the simplest unit of an element. Atoms that loose or gain electrons are called ions. Positively charged ions are called cations. Negatively charged ions are called anions. All atoms have a nucleus, which has protons and neutrons present. Protons are positively charged particles found within the nucleus. Neutrons do not carry a charge. The total of neutrons and protons is the mass number. The atomic number is the number of protons found in an atom. One mole of that element is the weight of the element required to equal its atomic weight. A compound is when 2 elements are found together in a definite ratio. The term molecule is a unit of two or more atoms that are bonded together. Avogadro's number 6.02×10^{23} is the number of molecules in one mole of that element.

Atoms can share electrons to bond called a covalent bond, or they can transfer electrons to another atom to form an ionic bond. In addition, a polar bond may be performed between substances in situations that a covalent or ionic bond is not desired. Compounds with various structures, but the same shape are called isomers.

Substances can exist in various states of matter. The three common states of matter are solid, liquid, and gas. Water can exist in all three forms. At 0 degrees Celsius water is a solid. At 100 degrees Celsius water becomes a gas. In solid form the molecules of water are moving very slowly. In liquid form the molecules of water are moving at a faster pace, and in gas form are highly excited. Converting liquid into a gas is known as evaporation. Converting gas into a liquid is known as condensation. Due to the fact that liquids and gases flow easily they are known as fluids. Transfer of a solid into a gas without going through the liquid state is known as sublimation.

Energy taken in or given off during reactions is measured as heat. Heat can be measured in various units. Units include: joule-.239 calories, calorie-degree of energy required to raise one gram of water at 14.5 Celsius degrees by a single degree of Celsius.

Solutions

The concept of solvent and solute are applicable to gases, liquids and solids. A solvent is the host substance and the solute is the substance that is can be dissolved in the solvent. A solution is a mixture with same composition made of 2 or more substances. A solution that contains the maximum amount of solute is called a saturated solution. A heterogenous mixture is a solution that contains unequal distribution of solvents in the solution. A physical change is a change in the state of matter. A chemical change is a change in the chemical composition of a compound.

When discussing acid and base relationships. An acid is substance that increases the hydrogen ion concentration in water. A base is a substance that increases the hydroxide ion count in water. A chemical reaction identifies a relationship between reactants and products. Products will be formed during a reaction and identified on the right side of the equation. Catalysts can be used to speed up a reaction or cause a reaction, however they are never destroyed.

Thermodynamics

Endothermic reactions are reactions that absorb energy. Exothermic reactions are reactions that give off energy/heat.

1st Law of Thermodynamics-energy is conserved with every process.
2nd Law of Thermodynamics-the total entropy of a chemical system and that of its area always increases if the chemical or physical change is spontaneous.
Entropy is defined as the quantity of disorder in a chemical environment.
Celsius to Fahrenheit Conversion

Fahrenheit (K) = Celsius degree +273.15

Fahrenheit (K) = (9/5K (Celsius)) +32

Kinetic Theory of Energy- all atoms are in constant motion

Gases obey the following laws:

Charles law (Gay Lussac's law)-volume of a gas varies indirectly with temperature with pressure constant.
V/T = constant

Boyle's law-volume of a gas varies inversely with pressure if temperature is constant.
The two common units of Pressure (P) are atmosphere and Mercury millimeters.
1 atm = 760 mm Hg
PV = constant

Avogadro's law –equal volumes of all gases contain the same number of molecules.
Avogadro's number- 6.02×10^{23}.

Ideal Gas Equation
PV = nRT

Newton's Laws of Motion

1st Law- (Law of Inertia) - A moving object will resist any change in velocity. A resting object with resist any change to begin moving.
2nd Law- (Force = Mass x Acceleration, F=ma) – The force of object in motion is equal to the mass of the object and the acceleration of the object.
Force can be defined in terms of newtons (N).

3rd Law- Greater force must be applied to create movement. A reaction force is generated when another force is applied to an object. The greater force will determine if movement is to occur.

Velocity is the rate of change of position. Acceleration is the rate of change of velocity.

Waves

Wavelength- the distance between the highest points of a wave
Amplitude- half of the height of a wave, from the top of a crest to the bottom of a trough

Key Formulas

Momentum = Mass x Velocity

Acceleration = $\dfrac{\text{Change in Velocity}}{\text{Total Time}}$

Speed = $\dfrac{\text{Distance}}{\text{Time}}$

Work=Force x Distance

Power= $\dfrac{F \times D}{T}$

Power= Voltage x Current
Watts=Voltage x Amperes

Ohm's law, V = I*R

I = current
V = potential difference
R = resistance

Backtrack for Units

When faced with a problem that you don't know the formula for, simply solve for the units in the answer choices. The units in the answer choices are your key to understanding what mathematical relationship exists between the numbers given in the question.

Example: A 600 Hz sound wave has a velocity of 160 m/s. What is the wavelength of this sound wave?

Even if you do not know the formula for wavelengths, you can backtrack to get the answer by using the units in the answer choices. The answer choices are:

    A. 0.17 m
    B. 0.27 m
    C. 0.35 m
    D. 0.48 m

You know that Hz is equal to 1/s. To get an answer in m, when working with a m/s and a 1/s from the problem, you must divide the m/s by 1/s, which will leave an answer in meters or m. Therefore (160 m/s) / (600 1/s) = .27 m, making choice B correct.

Don't Fall for the Obvious

When in doubt of the answer, it is easy to go with what you are familiar with. If you recognize only one term in four answer choices, you may be inclined to guess at that term. Be careful though, and don't go with familiar answers simply because they are familiar.

Example: Changing the temperature of the solution to 373K would most likely result in:

    A. boiling the solution
    B. freezing the solution
    C. dissolving the compound
    D. saturating the solution

You know that 373K is the boiling point of pure water. Therefore choice A is familiar, because you have a mental link between the temperature 373K and the word "boiling". If you are unsure of the correct answer, you may decide upon choice A simply because of its familiarity. Don't be deceived though. Think through the other answer choices before making your final selection. Just because you have a mental link between two terms, doesn't make an answer choice correct.

Milk the Question

Some of the questions may throw you completely off. They might deal with a subject you have not been exposed to, or one that you haven't reviewed in years. While your lack of knowledge about the subject will be a hindrance, the question itself can give you many clues that will help you find the correct answer. Read the question carefully, and look for clues. Watch particularly for adjectives and nouns describing difficult terms or words that you don't recognize. Regardless of if you understand a word or not, replacing it with the synonyms used for it in the question may help you to understand what the questions are asking.

Example: A bacteriophage is a virus that infects bacteria….

While you may not know much information concerning the characteristics of a bacteriophage, the fifth word into the sentence told you that a bacteriophage is a virus. Whenever a question asks about a bacteriophage, you can mentally replace the word "bacteriophage" with the word "virus". Your more general knowledge of viruses will enable you to answer the question intelligibly.

Look carefully for these descriptive synonyms (nouns) and adjectives and use them to help you understand the difficult terms. Rather than wracking your mind about specific detail information concerning a difficult term in the question, use the more general description or synonym provided to make it easier for you.

Work Fast

Since you have 60 questions to answer in only 60 minutes, that means that you have 1 minute to spend per question. This section faces a greater time crunch that any other test you will take on the PSB H.O. exam, for though the Verbal Test also has a 1 minute per question time restriction, the questions in the Science Test may sometimes have calculations associated with them that could require more time. While the Mathematics Test allows 1.5 minutes for these calculation questions, there is no such luxury for the Science Test. Therefore, if you are stuck on one word, don't waste too much time. Eliminate the answers you could bet a quick $5 on and then pick the first one that remains. You can make a note in your book and if you have time you can always come back, but don't waste your time. You have to work fast!

Random Tips

- On fact questions that require choosing between numbers, don't guess the smallest or largest choice unless you're sure of the answer (remember- "sure" means you would bet $5 on it).
- For questions that you're not clear on the answer, use the process of elimination. Weed out the answer choices that you know are wrong before choosing an answer.
- Don't fall for "bizarre" choices, mentioning things that are not relevant to the passage. Also avoid answers that sound "smart." Again, if you're willing to bet $5, ignore the tips and go with your bet.

Part V. – Vocational Adjustment Index

This is a mini-test that evaluates your opinions and attitudes related to the nursing profession and practice as a professional. You cannot prepare for this section of the PSB-H.O. exam. You will be asked questions on quality of care, delivery of services, and patient rights. Moreover, the goal of this mini-test is to determine your opinions about professional care. If you answer with "extreme" points of view, you will not be scored well on this assessment.

Special Report: Practice Test

Please use the online spelling review links for spelling practice. This practice test does not contain practice questions for the part I -form relationships test, or the vocational adjustment index. The vocational adjustment index covers questions that only ask your opinions about professional practice. In addition, the form relationship principles reviewed in this guide cover the necessary skills that can be applied to a vast variety of objects for analysis.

Part I- Vocabulary Review

1. The data in the graph exhibited an *aberration*.
   Aberration means:

   A: deviation from course
   B: linear appearance
   C: inverted appearance
   D: circular theme

2. The prince *abjured* the ambassador.
   Abjured means:

   A: congratulated
   B: renounced
   C: relieved
   D: fired

3. The chemist attempted to practice *alchemy*.
   Alchemy means:

   A: turning metal into gold
   B: separating ions
   C: fusion
   D: isolating chemical components

4. The man at the bar was *belligerent*.
   Belligerent means:

   A: friendly
   B: courteous
   C: angry
   D: talkative

5. The ships formed a *blockade* near the mouth of the Mississippi River.

Blockade means:

A: prevent passage
B: fishing convoy
C: whaling expedition
D: zigzag formation

6. The men erected a *bulwark* near the opening.
    Bulwark means:

A: trap
B: obstacle
C: barn
D: runway

7. The group embarked on a *clandestine* operation.
    Clandestine means:

A: environmental expedition
B: shipping adventure
C: scary
D: secretive

8. The agent of the government was *choleric*.
    Choleric means:

A: easily provoked
B: undercover
C: cooperative
D: late

9. Some members of the organization broke away and created a grass roots *caucus*.
    Caucus means:

A: group with political aims
B: environmental group
C: management organization
D: religious movement

10. The facts were open to *conjecture*.
    Conjecture means:

A: discussion
B: guessing
C: argument

D: public

11. The news anchor attempted to *disseminate* the story.
    Disseminate means:

A: to convey
B: to deny
C: to rebuke
D: to review

12. The stockpiles for the occupation began to *dwindle*.
    Dwindle means:

A: to increase
B: to decrease
C: to rot
D: to be self-limiting

13. The chemicals began to *effervesce*.
    Effervesce means:

A: to combine
B: to catalyze
C: to break down
D: to bubble up

14. The witness began to *evince* critical details.
    Evince means:

A: to hide
B: to cover secretly
C: exaggerate
D: to make manifest

15. The front line troops began to *extricate* from the enemy.
    Extricate means:

A: confront
B: surrender
C: disentangle
D: deploy

16. The congressman from Ohio started a *filibuster*.
    Filibuster means:

A: bill
B: congressional investigation
C: an attempt to disrupt legislation
D: program related to welfare

17. The soldier showed *fortitude* during the engagement with the enemy.
    Fortitude means:

A: patient courage
B: willingness for action
C: endurance
D: professionalism

18. The southern lady was *genteel* when hosting northern businessmen.
    Genteel means:

A: rude
B: refined
C: reserved
D: resentful

19. The lawyer launched into a *harangue* when speaking to the witness.
    Harangue means:

A: discussion
B: monologue
C: dialogue
D: tirade

20. Some believe our destinies are *immutable*.
    Immutable means:

A: professional
B: conversational
C: unchangeable
D: unerring

21. The baby was diagnosed with *jaundice*.
    Jaundice means:

A: yellowing condition
B: condition of glucose intolerance
C: condition of nutritional deficiency
D: condition of dermatitis

22. The criminal was known for his *knavery*.
    Knavery means:

A: quickness
B: light-footedness
C: burglary ability
D: deceitfulness

23. The patient exhibited signs of *languor*.
    Languor means:

A: confusion
B: anxiety
C: depression
D: deceitfulness

24. The Romans were able to *macadamize* a large portion of the Italian peninsula.
    Macadamize means:

A: to pave
B: to supply
C: to connect
D: to protect

25. The patient's lower extremity began to show signs of *necrosis*.
    Necrosis means:

A: maceration
B: tissue death
C: induration
D: redness

26. The traffic official began to *obviate* the construction.
    Obviate means:

A: clear away
B: identify
C: reproduce
D: delegate

27. The general *presaged* the battle plan to his subordinate officers.
    Presaged means:

A: delegated
B: clarified

- 63 -

C: foretold
D: introduced

28. The orange grove was under *quarantine*, because of a local virus.
    Quarantine means:

A: pressure
B: demolition
C: reconstruction
D: isolation

29. The defendant was asked to *remunerate* the damage he caused during the robbery.
    Remunerate means:

A: reconstruct
B: renounce
C: pay for
D: repeat

30. The welding machine *scintillated* into the dark shop.
    Scintillated means:

A: emitted gases
B: emitted light
C: emitted fumes
D: emitted noise

31. The mission was *surreptitious* in nature.
    Surreptitious means:

A: transforming
B: dangerous
C: invasive
D: secret

32. The desert conditions were *torrid* for the Israeli division operating in the Sinai.
    Torrid means:

A: excessively hot
B: aggravating
C: lukewarm
D: inhospitable

33. The adventurer left with a feeling of *trepidation*.

Trepidation means:

A: uncertainty
B: extreme depression
C: ambivalence
D: fearfulness

34. The fish exhibited an *unctuous* appearance at the fish market.
    Unctuous means:

A: fresh
B: dirty
C: oily
D: lucid

35. The venal politician preyed upon his constituents during his time in office.
    Venal means:

A: barbaric
B: current
C: ambivalent
D: corrupt

Part I - Mathematics Review
(no calculator)

36.   897.54 – 48.39 =

A: 849.15
B: 813.15
C: 859.15
D: 814.15

37.   1053.33 – 545.69 =

A: 519.64
B: 517.54
C: 508.64
D: 507.64

38.   893.42 + 82.77 =

A: 976.09
B: 976.29
C: 986.19

D: 976.19

39.   94.31 + 973.37 =

A: 1067.68
B: 1167.68
C: 1067.78
D: 1167.78

40.   A senior paid $3.47, $9.50 and $2.50 for lunch during a basketball
       tournament. What was the average amount he paid over three days?

A: $5.18
B: $5.25
C: $5.16
D: $5.37

41.   89.35 x 32.75 =

A: 2826.23
B: 2925.31
C: 2926.21
D: 2837.41

42.   Using the following equation, solve for (x). $3x - 4y = 25$ and $(y)=2$

A: x =10
B: x = 11
C: x = 12
D: x = 13

43.   Using the following equation, solve for (y). $5y - 3x = 24$ and $(x) = 7$

A: y = 8
B: y = 9
C: y = 10
D: y = 11

44.   The amount of %5 was the local tax at an auction. An armoire was purchased
       for $340.32. What was the additional tax charged on the armoire?

A: $15.82
B: $16.02
C: $16.39
D: $17.02

45.   894 + ((3)(12)) =

A: 730
B: 932
C: 930
D: 945

46.   Round to the nearest 2 decimal places, 892/15 =

A: 60.47
B: 59.47
C: 62.57
D: 59.57

47.   Round to the nearest 2 decimal places, 999.52/13 =

A: 76.89
B: 76.97
C: 86.87
D: 86.97

48.   Round to the nearest 2 decimal places, 9.42/3.47 =

A: 2.63
B: 2.71
C: 2.81
D: 2.94

49.   Jonathan Edwards ate 8.32 lbs. of food over 3 days. What was his average
        intake?

A: 2.66 lbs.
B: 2.77 lbs.
C: 2.87 lbs.
D: 2.97 lbs.

50.   Which of the following decimals equals 9.47%?

A: .000947
B: .00947
C: .0947
D: .9470

51.   .10 equals which of the following fractions?

A: 1/100
B: 1/10
C: 1/50
D: 1/5

52.   What is the area of a rectangle with sides 34 meters and 12 meters?

A: 408
B: 2.83
C: 22
D: 40.8

53.   The standard ratio of (number of treatments) and (total mL dose) are 3.5 to 2 mL. If only 2 treatments are given, how many total mL doses are given?

A: 1.58 mL
B: 2.34 mL
C: 1.14 mL
D: 2.58 mL

54.   If one side of a triangle equals 4 inches and the second side equals 5 inches, what does the third side equal?

A: 9 inches
B: 1 inches
C: 6.4 inches
D: 4.6 inches

55.   If x=75 + 0, and y= (75)(0), then

A: x>y
B: x=y
C: x<y
D: x+y = 0

56.   If x=3, the $x^2+x=$

A: 9
B: 15
C: 12
D: 10

57.   If a=4 and b=5, then a $(a^2+b)=$

- 68 -

A: 52
B: 84
C: 62
D: 64

58.   If x= ¼, y=1/2, and z= 2/3, then x + y- z =

A: 1/8
B: 2/9
C: 1/12
D: 2/5

59.   If x= ½, y=1/3, z=3/8, then x(y-z)=

A: 1/48
B: -1/48
C: 1/64
D: -1/64

60:     If 2/3 cup of oil is needed for a cake recipe, and you have ¼ cup of oil. How much more do you need?

A: 1/2
B: 2/7
C: 3/8
D: 5/12

61:     8 ¾ + 6 ½ =

A: 32
B: 15 ¼
C: 14 ½
D: 17 ¾

62.   A senior citizen was billed $ 3.85 for a long-distance phone call. The first 10 minutes cost $3.50, and 35 cents was charged for each additional minute. How long was the telephone call?

A: 17 minutes
B: 20 minutes
C: 15 minutes
D: 11 minutes

63.   A ½ cup of skim milk is 45 calories. Approximately how may calories would ¾ cup of skim milk provide?

A: 67 ½
B: 68
C: 76 ½
D: 60

64. $10b = 5a - 15$. If $a = 3$, then $b =$

A: 7
B: 5
C: 1
D: 0

65. $(5 \times 4) \div (2 \times 2) =$

A: 6
B: 7.2
C: 5
D: 4

66.   Which of these numbers is a prime number?

A: 12
B: 4
C: 15
D: 11

67.   If 12 members of a weight loss club are female, there are 23 members. Approximately what percentage is male?

A: 59%
B: 48%
C: 36%
D: 44%

68. A person travels an average of 57 miles daily, and this morning he traveled 14 miles. What percentage of his daily average of mile traveled did he travel this morning?

A: 25%
B: 22%
C: 27%
D: 32%

69.   75 is 60% of what number?

A: 130
B: 125
C: 45
D: 145

70.   If a student invests $3000 of his student loan and receives 400 dollars in Interest, over a 4-year period. What is his average yearly interest rate?

A: 3.3%
B: 2.1%
C: 5%
D: 4.2%

Part III- Reading Comprehension Test

See bonus download- the last page of this document for complete reading comprehension practice tests.

Part IV- Science Review

71.   The heart is divided into __ chambers.

A: 2
B: 3
C: 4
D: 5

72.   Blood leaves the right ventricle and goes to the ____.

A: lungs
B: kidneys
C: right atrium
D: arterial circulation to the body

73.   Which of the following does not help determine heart rate?

A: body temperature
B: physical activity
C: concentration of ions
D: anaerobic cellular metabolism

74.   Which of the following is not considered a layer of the heart?

A: epicardium
B: endocarcium
C: myocardium
D: vasocardium

75.   The hormone _____ can promote increased blood volume, and increased blood pressure.

A: estrogen
B: testosterone
C: aldosterone
D: dopamine

76.   Which of the following terms matches the definition: an abnormally slow heartbeat.

A: tachycardia
B: bradycardia
C: fibrillation
D: myocardial infarct

77.   Blood is made of approximate ___% hematocrit and ____55% plasma.

A: 45, 55
B: 55, 45
C: 75, 25
D: 25, 75

78.   The right lung has ___ lobes and the left lung has ___ lobes.

A: 2, 3
B: 3, 2
C: 4, 2
D: 2, 4

79.   Aerobic respiration in cells occurs in the _____.

A: cytoplasm
B: nucleus
C: mitochondria
D: cell membrane

80.   Which of the following terms matches the definition: collapse of a lung.

A: anoxia
B: atelectasis
C: dyspnea
D: hypercapnia

81.   The central nervous system is composed of the _____ and the _____.

A: brain, spinal cord
B: brain, peripheral nerves
C: spinal cord, peripheral nerves
D: spinal cord, musculature system

82.   The brain is made of _____ lobes.

A: 2
B: 3
C: 4
D: 5

83.   _____ is a state of equilibrium within tissues.

A: peristalsis
B: somatitis
C: homeostasis
D: synergy

84.   _____ is a state of inflammation of the mouth.

A: diverticulitis
B: hepatitis
C: enteritis
D: somatitis

85.   _____ is the most important male hormone

A: estrogen
B: aldosterone
C: progesterone
D: testosterone

86.   Which of the following functions are not related to the kidneys?

A: filtration
B: bile production
C: secretion

- 73 -

D: re-absorption

87. Which of the following terms matches the definition: uncontrolled urination.

A: enuresis
B: dieuretic
C: pyuria
D: ureteritis

88. Auditory impulses are interpreted in the _____ lobes.

A: frontal
B: parietal
C: temporal
D: occipital

89. The outer layer of the eye is the ____.

A: cornea
B: sclera
C: retina
D: rods

90. The inner layer of the eye is the ____.

A: cornea
B: sclera
C: retina
D: rods

91. Which of the following elements are not halogens?

A: Chlorine
B: Bromide
C: Iodine
D: Cesium

92. The horizontal rows of the periodic table are called _____.

A: periods
B: columns
C: rows
D: families

93 A/an ____ is the simplest unit of an element.

A: atom
B: molecule
C: electron
D: neutron

94.   Compounds with various structures, but the same shape are called _____.

A: polar compounds
B: isomers
C: variables
D: transient compounds

95.   Converting gas into a liquid is known as _____.

A: evaporation
B: transitioning
C: condensation
D: sublimation

96.   Which of the following terms matches the definition: the volume of a gas varies indirectly with temperature with pressure constant.

A: Boyle's law
B: Charles law
C: Johnson's law
D: Avogadro's law

97.   Which of the following terms matches the definition: energy is conserved with every process.

A: 1st Law of Thermodynamics
B: 2nd Law of Thermodynamics
C: 3rd Law of Thermodynamics
D: 4th Law of Thermodynamics

98.   An acid is a substance that increases the _____ count in water.

A: chloride ion
B: hydroxide ion
C: hydrogen ion
D: oxygen

99.   Which of the following is not true of reaction catalysts potential?

A: speed up a reaction
B: cause a reaction
C: never destroyed
D: always found on the right side of an equation

100.   Using the 2nd Law of Newton identify the formula that is applicable.

A: F=ma
B: Speed = $\dfrac{\text{Distance}}{\text{Time}}$

C: Power = $\dfrac{F \times D}{T}$

D: Watts = Voltage x Amperes

1. A	35. D	69. B
2. B	36. A	70. A
3. A	37. D	71. C
4. C	38. D	72. A
5. A	39. A	73. D
6. B	40. C	74. D
7. D	41. C	75. C
8. A	42. B	76. B
9. A	43. B	77. A
10. B	44. D	78. B
11. A	45. C	79. C
12. B	46. B	80. B
13. D	47. A	81. A
14. D	48. B	82. C
15. C	49. B	83. C
16. C	50. C	84. D
17. A	51. B	85. D
18. B	52. A	86. B
19. D	53. C	87. A
20. C	54. C	88. C
21. A	55. A	89. B
22. D	56. C	90. C
23. C	57. B	91. D
24. A	58. C	92. A
25. B	59. B	93. A
26. A	60. D	94. B
27. C	61. B	95. C
28. D	62. D	96. B
29. C	63. A	97. A
30. B	64. D	98. C
31. D	65. C	99. D
32. A	66. D	100. A
33. D	67. B	
34. C	68. A	

Special Report: PSB H.O. Secrets in Action

Sample Question from the Mathematics Test:

Three coins are tossed up in the air. What is the probability that two of them will land heads and one will land tails?

A. 0
B. 1/8
C. 1/4
D. 3/8

Let's look at a few different methods and steps to solving this problem.

1. Reduction and Division

Quickly eliminate the probabilities that you immediately know. You know to roll all heads is a 1/8 probability, and to roll all tails is a 1/8 probability. Since there are in total 8/8 probabilities, you can subtract those two out, leaving you with 8/8 – 1/8 – 1/8 = 6/8. So after eliminating the possibilities of getting all heads or all tails, you're left with 6/8 probability. Because there are only three coins, all other combinations are going to involve one of either head or tail, and two of the other. All other combinations will either be 2 heads and 1 tail, or 2 tails and 1 head. Those remaining combinations both have the same chance of occurring, meaning that you can just cut the remaining 6/8 probability in half, leaving you with a 3/8ths chance that there will be 2 heads and 1 tail, and another 3/8ths chance that there will be 2 tails and 1 head, making choice D correct.

2. Run Through the Possibilities for that Outcome

You know that you have to have two heads and one tail for the three coins. There are only so many combinations, so quickly run through them all.

You could have:
H, H, H
H, H, T
H, T, H
T, H, H
T, T, H
T, H, T
H, T, T
T, T, T

Reviewing these choices, you can see that three of the eight have two heads and one tail, making choice D correct.

3. Fill in the Blanks with Symbology and Odds

Many probability problems can be solved by drawing blanks on a piece of scratch paper (or making mental notes) for each object used in the problem, then filling in probabilities and multiplying them out. In this case, since there are three coins being flipped, draw three blanks. In the first blank, put an "H" and over it write "1/2". This represents the case where the first coin is flipped as heads. In that case (where the first coin comes up heads), one of the other two coins must come up tails and one must come up heads to fulfill the criteria posed in the problem (2 heads and 1 tail). In the second blank, put a "1" or "1/1". This is because it doesn't matter what is flipped for the second coin, so long as the first coin is heads. In the third blank, put a "1/2". This is because the third coin must be the exact opposite of whatever is in the second blank. Half the time the third coin will be the same as the second coin, and half the time the third coin will be the opposite, hence the "1/2". Now multiply out the odds. There is a half chance that the first coin will come up "heads", then it doesn't matter for the second coin, then there is a half chance that the third coin will be the opposite of the second coin, which will give the desired result of 2 heads and 1 tail. So, that gives 1/2*1/1*1/2 = 1/4.

But, now you must calculate the probabilities that result if the first coin is flipped tails. So draw another group of three blanks. In the first blank, put a "T" and over it write "1/2". This represents the case where the first coin is flipped as tails. In that case (where the first coin comes up tails), both of the other two coins must come up heads to fulfill the criteria posed in the problem. In the second blank, put an "H" and over it write "1/2". In the third blank, put an "H" and over it write "1/2". Now multiply out the odds. There is a half chance that the first coin will come up "tails", then there is a half chance that the second coin will be heads, and a half chance that the third coin will be heads. So, that gives 1/2*1/2*1/2 = 1/8.

Now, add those two probabilities together. If you flip heads with the first coin, there is a 1/4 chance of ultimately meeting the problem's criteria. If you flip tails with the first coin, there is a 1/8 chance of ultimately meeting the problem's criteria. So, that gives 1/4 + 1/8 = 2/8 + 1/8 = 3/8, which makes choice D correct.

Sample Question from the Reading Comprehension Test:

Mark Twain was well aware of his celebrity. He was among the first authors to employ a clipping service to track press coverage of himself, and it was not unusual for him to issue his own press statements if he wanted to influence or "spin" coverage of a particular story. The celebrity Twain achieved during his last ten years still reverberates today. Nearly all of his most popular novels were published before 1890, long before his hair grayed or he began to wear his famous white suit in public. We appreciate the author but seem to remember the celebrity.

Based on the passage above, Mark Twain seemed interested in:

    A. maintaining his celebrity
    B. selling more of his books
    C. hiding his private life
    D. gaining popularity

Let's look at a couple of different methods of solving this problem.

1. Identify the key words in each answer choice. These are the nouns and verbs that are the most important words in the answer choice.

A. maintaining, celebrity
B. selling, books
C. hiding, life
D. gaining, popularity

Now try to match up each of the key words with the passage and see where they fit. You're trying to find synonyms and/or exact replication between the key words in the answer choices and key words in the passage.

A. maintaining – no matches; celebrity – matches in sentences 1, 3, and 5
B. selling – no matches; books – matches with "novels" in sentence 4.
C. hiding – no matches; life – no matches
D. gaining – no matches; popularity –matches with "celebrity" in sentences 1, 3, and
    5, because they can be synonyms

At this point there are only two choices that have more than one match, choices A and D, and they both have the same number of matches, and with the same word in the passage, which is the word "celebrity" in the passage. This is a good sign, because the test writers will often write two answer choices that are close. Having two answer choices pointing towards the same key word is a strong indicator that those key words hold the "key" to finding the right answer.

Now let's compare choice A and D and the unmatched key words. Choice A still has "maintaining" which doesn't have a clear match, while choice D has "gaining" which doesn't have a clear match. While neither of those have clear matches in the passage, ask yourself what are the best arguments that would support any kind of connection with either of those two words.

"Maintaining" makes sense when you consider that Twain was interested in tracking his press coverage and that he was actively managing the "spin" of certain stories.

"Gaining" makes sense when you consider that Twain was actively issuing his own press releases, however one key point to remember is that he was only issuing these press releases after another story was already in existence.

Since Twain's press releases were not being released in a news vacuum, but rather as a response mechanism to ensure control over the angle of a story, his releases were more to *maintain* control over his image, rather than *gain* an image in the first place.

Furthermore, when comparing the terms "popularity" and "celebrity", there are similarities between the words, but in referring back to the passage, it is clear that "celebrity" has a stronger connection to the passage, being the exact word used three times in the passage.

Since "celebrity" has a stronger match than "popularity" and "maintaining" makes more sense than "gaining," it is clear that choice A is correct.

2. Use a process of elimination.

A. maintaining his celebrity – The passage discusses how Mark Twain was both aware of his celebrity status and would take steps to ensure that he got the proper coverage in any news story and maintained the image he desired. This is the correct answer.

B. selling more of his books – Mark Twain's novels are mentioned for their popularity and while common sense would dictate that he would be interested in selling more of his books, the passage makes no mention of him doing anything to promote sales.

C. hiding his private life – While the passage demonstrates that Mark Twain was keenly interested in how the public viewed his life, it does not indicate that he cared about hiding his private life, not even mentioning his life outside of the public eye. The passage deals with how he was seen by the public.

D. gaining popularity – At first, this sounds like a good answer choice, because Mark Twain's popularity is mentioned several times. The main difference though is that he wasn't trying to gain popularity, but simply ensuring that the popularity he had was not distorted by bad press.

.

Sample Question from the Natural Science Test:

Table 1

Length of 0.10 mm diameter aluminum wire (m)	Resistance (ohms) at 20° C
1	3.55
2	7.10
4	14.20
10	35.50

Based on the information in Table 1, one would predict that a 20 m length of aluminum wire with a 0.10 mm diameter would have a resistance of:

A. 16 ohms
B. 25 ohms
C. 34 ohms
D. 71 ohms

Let's look at a few different methods and steps to solving this problem.

1. Create a Proportion or Ratio

The first way you could approach this problem is by setting up a proportion or ratio. You will find that many of the problems on the PSB H.O. exam can be solved using this simple technique. Usually whenever you have a given pair of numbers (this number goes with that number) and you are given a third number and asked to find what number would be its match, then you have a problem that can be converted into an easy proportion or ratio.

In this case you can take any of the pairs of numbers from Table 1. As an example, let's choose the second set of numbers (2 m and 7.10 ohms).

Form a question with the information you have at your disposal: 2 meters goes to 7.10 ohms as 20 meters (from the question) goes to which resistance?

From your ratio: 2m/7.10 ohms = 20m/x
"x" is used as the missing number that you will solve for.

Cross multiplication provides us with 2*x = 7.10*20 or 2x = 142.

Dividing both sides by 2 gives us 2x/2 = 142/2 or x = 71, making choice D correct.

2. Use Algebra

The question is asking for the resistance of a 20 m length of wire. The resistance is a function of the length of the wire, so you know that you could probably set up an algebra problem that would have 20 multiplied by some factor "x" that would give you your answer.

So, now you have 20*x = ?

But what exactly is "x"? If 20*x would give you the resistance of a 20 foot piece of wire, than 1*x would give you the resistance of a 1 foot piece of wire. Remember though, the table already told you the resistance of a 1 foot piece of wire – it's 3.55 ohms.

So, if 1*x = 3.55 ohms, then solving for "x" gives you x = 3.55 ohms.

Plugging your solution for "x" back into your initial equation of 20*x = ?, you now have 20*3.55 ohms = 71 ohms, making choice D correct.

3. Look for a Pattern

Much of the time you can get by with just looking for patterns on problems that provide you with a lot of different numbers. In this case, consider the provided table.

1 – 3.55
2 – 7.10
4 – 14.20
10 – 35.50

What patterns do you see in the above number sequences. It appears that when the number in the first column doubled from 1 to 2, the numbers in the second column doubled as well, going from 3.55 to 7.10. Further inspection shows that when the numbers in the first column doubled from 2 to 4, the numbers in the second column doubled again, going from 7.10 to 14.20. Now you've got a pattern, when the first column of numbers doubles, so does the second column.

Since the question asked about a resistance of 20, you should recognize that 20 is the double of 10. Since a length of 10 meant a resistance of 35.50 ohms, then doubling the length of 10 should double the resistance, making 71 ohms, or choice D, correct.

4. Use Logic

A method that works even faster than finding patterns or setting up equations is using simple logic. It appears that as the first number (the length of the wire) gets larger, so does the second number (the resistance).

Since the length of 10 (the largest length wire in the provided table) has a corresponding resistance of 35.50, then another length (such as 20 in the question) should have a length greater than 35.50. As you inspect the answer choices, there is only one answer choice that is greater than 35.50, which is choice D, making it correct.

Special Report: Which PSB-Exam Study Guides and Practice Tests Are Worth Your Time

We believe the following guides present uncommon value to our customers who wish to "really study" for the PSB H.O. exam. While our manual teaches some valuable tricks and tips that no one else covers, learning the basic coursework tested on the PSB H.O. exam is also helpful, though more time consuming.

Practice Tests

To our knowledge the official PSB organization does not offer practice questions for students, and no other author has written a specific book to cover this exam. If you are aware of additional specific review questions please let us know.

{The NLN (National League for Nursing) sponsors the RN pre-entrance exam, which has valuable practice although it is not associated directly with PSB test and is a separate test.} It will not match up in format as well as our practice questions.

Pre-entrance exam Information

http://www.nln.org/

(Call the National League for Nursing Office at 1-800-669-9656 to order)

Study Guide

Review Guide for NLN RN Pre-Entrance Exam...

http://www.amazon.com/exec/obidos/tg/detail/-/0763724866/qid=1081354386/sr=1-1/ref=sr_1_1/002-0119763-4408008?v=glance&s=books

Appendix: Area, Volume, Surface Area Formulas

These are valuable to memorize for the Mathematics Test:

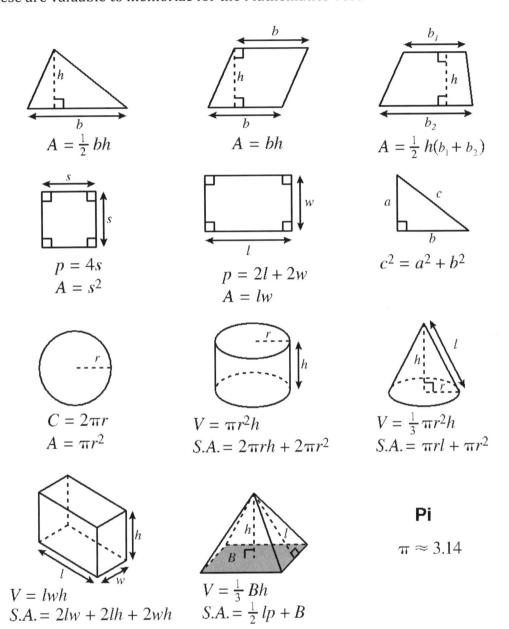

$A = \frac{1}{2} bh$

$A = bh$

$A = \frac{1}{2} h(b_1 + b_2)$

$p = 4s$
$A = s^2$

$p = 2l + 2w$
$A = lw$

$c^2 = a^2 + b^2$

$C = 2\pi r$
$A = \pi r^2$

$V = \pi r^2 h$
$S.A. = 2\pi rh + 2\pi r^2$

$V = \frac{1}{3} \pi r^2 h$
$S.A. = \pi rl + \pi r^2$

$V = lwh$
$S.A. = 2lw + 2lh + 2wh$

$V = \frac{1}{3} Bh$
$S.A. = \frac{1}{2} lp + B$

Pi

$\pi \approx 3.14$

Special Report: Musculature/Innervation Review of the Arm and Back

Muscle	Origin	Insertion	Nerve
Trapezius	Ext. Occipit Protuberance, Spines of T Vertebrae	Lateral Clavicle, Spine of the Scapula	Spinal Accessory Nerve CN XI
Latissimus Dorsi	Spines of Lower 6 T Vertebrae, Iliac Crest and Lower 4 Ribs	Bicipital Groove	Thoracodorsal
Levator Scapulae	Transverse Process of C1-C4	Upper Medial Border of Scapula	Dorsal Scapula
Rhomboid Major	Spinous Process of T2-T5	Medial Border Scapula Below Spine	Dorsal Scapular
Rhomboid Minor	Spinous Process of C7-T1	Medial Border Scapula Opp. Spine	Dorsal Scapular
Teres Major	Lateral Dorsal Inferior Angle of Scapula	Bicipital Groove	Lower Subscapular
Teres Minor	Lateral Scapula 2/3 way down	Greater Tubercle of Humerus	Axillary
Deltoid	Lateral 1/3 Clavicle and Acromion Process, Spine of the Scapula	Deltoid Tuberosity	Axillary
Supraspinatus	Supraspinatus Fossa	Greater Tubercle of Humerus	Suprascapular
Infraspinatus	Infaspinatus Fossa	Greater Tubercle of Humerus	Suprascapular
Subscapularis	Subscapular Fossa	Lesser Tubercle of Humerus	Upper and lower Subscapular
Serratus Anterior	Slips of Upper 8-9 Ribs	Ventral-Medial Border Scapula	Long Thoracic
Subclavius	Inferior Surface of the Clavicle	First Rib	Nerve to the Subclavius
Pectoralis Major	Medial ½ clavicle and Side of	Bicipital Groove	Medial and Lateral Pectoral

	Sternum		
Pectoralis Minor	Ribs 3,4,5 or 2,3,4	Coracoid Process	Medial Pectoral
Biceps Branchii	Supraglenoid Tubercle	Posterior Margin of Radial Tuberosity	Musculocutaneous
Coracobrachialis	Coracoid Process	Medial Humerus at Deltoid Tuberosity Level	Musculocutaneous
Brachialis	Anterior-Lateral ½ of Humerus	Ulnar Tuberosity and Coronoid Process	Musculocutaneous
Triceps Brachii	Infraglenoid Tubercle, Below and Medial to the Radial Groove	Olecranon Process	Radial
Anconeus	Posterior, Lateral Humeral Condyle	Upper Posterior Ulna	Radial
Brachioradialis	Lateral Supracondylar Ridge of Humerus	Radial Styloid Process	Radial
Pronator Teres	Medial Epicondyle and Supracondylar Ridge	½ Way Down on Lateral Radius	Median
Pronator Quadratus	Distal-Medial Ulna	Distal-Lateral Radius	Anterior Interosseous

Musculature/Innervation Review of the Forearm

Muscle	Origin	Insertion	Nerve
Brachioradialis	Lateral Supracondylar Ridge of Humerus	Radial Styloid Process	Radial
Pronator Teres	Medial Epicondyle and Supracondylar Ridge	½ Way Down on Lateral Radius	Median
Pronator Quadratus	Distal-Medial Ulna	Distal-Lateral Radius	Anterior Interosseous
Supinator	Lateral Epicondyle of Humerus	Upper ½ Lateral, Posterior Radius	Posterior Inter-Deep Radial
Flexor Carpi Radialis	Medial Epicondyle of Humerus	2nd and 3rd Metacarpal	Median
Flexor Carpi Ulnaris	Medial Epicondyle of Humerus	Pisiform, Hamate, 5th Metacarpal	Ulnar

Palmaris Longus	Medial Epicondyle of the Humerus	Palmar Aponeurosis and Flexor Retinaculum	Median
Flexor Digitorum Suerficialis	Medial Epicondyle, Radius, Ulna	Medial 4 Digits	Median
Flexor Digitorum Profundus	Ulna, Interosseous Membrane	Medial 4 Digits (distal part)	Median (lateral 2 digits), Ulnar (median 2 digits)
Flexor Pollicis Longus	Radius	Distal Phalanx (thumb)	Anterior Inter-Deep Median
Extensor Carpi Radialis Longus	Lateral Condyle and Supracondylar Ridge	2nd Metacarpal	Radial
Extensor Carpi Radialis Brevis	Lateral Epicondyle of Humerus	3rd Metacarpal	Posterior Inter-Deep Radial
Extensor Carpi Ulnaris	Lateral Epicondyle of Humerus	5th Metacarpal	Posterior Inter-Deep Radial
Extensor Digitorum	Lateral Epicondyle of Humerus	Extension Expansion Hood of Medial 4 Digits	Posterior Inter-Deep Radial
Extensor Digiti Minimi	Lateral Epicondyle of Humerus	Extension Expansion Hood of (little finger)	Posterior Inter-Deep Radial
Abductor Pollicis Longus	Posterior Radius and Ulna	Radial Side of 1st Metacarpal	Posterior Inter-Deep Radial
Extensor Indicis	Ulna and Interosseous Membrane	Extension Expansion Hood (index finger)	Posterior Inter-Deep Radial
Extensor Pollicis Longus	Ulna and Interosseous Membrane	Distal Phalanx (thumb)	Posterior Inter-Deep Radial
Extensor Pollicis Brevis	Radius	Proximal Phalanx (thumb)	Posterior Inter-Deep Radial

Musculature/Innervation Review of the Hand

Muscle	Origin	Insertion	Nerve
Adductor Policis	Capitate and Base of Adjacent Metacarpals	Proximal Phalanx (thumb)	Deep Branch of Ulnar
Lumbricals	Tendons of Flexor	Extension	Deep Branch Ulnar

	Digitorum Profundas	Expansion Hood of Medial 4 Digits	(medial 2 Ls), Median (lateral 2 Ls)
Dorsal Interosseous Muscles (4)	Sides of Metacarpals	Extension Expansion Hood of Digits 2-4	Deep Branch Ulnar
Palmar Interosseous (3)	Sides of Metacarpals	Extension Expansion Hood, Digits 2,4,5	Deep Branch Ulnar
Palmaris Brevis	Anterior Flexor Retinaculum and Palmar Aponeurosis	Skin-Ulnar Border of Hand	Superficial Ulnar
Abductor Pollicis Brevis	Flexor Retinaculum, Trapezium	Lateral Proximal Phalanx (thumb)	Median (thenar branch)
Flexor Pollicis Brevis	Flexor Retinaculum, Trapezium	Lateral Proximal Phalanx (thumb)	Median (thenar branch)
Opponens Pollicis	Flexor Retinaculum, Trapezium	Radial Border (1st Metacarpal)	Median (thenar branch)
Abductor Digiti Minimi	Flexor Retinaculum, Pisiform	Proximal Phalanx (little finger)	Deep Branch Ulnar
Flexor Digiti Minimi	Flexor Retinaculum, Hamate	Proximal Phalanx (little finger)	Deep Branch Ulnar
Opponens Digiti Minimi	Flexor Retinaculum, Hamate	Ulnar Medial Border (5th Metacarpal)	Deep Branch Ulnar

Musculature/Innervation Review of the Thigh

Muscle	Origin	Insertion	Nerve
Psoas Major	Bodies and Discs of T12-L5	Lesser Trochanter	L2,3
Psoas Minor	Bodies and Discs of T12 and L1	Pectineal Line of Superior Pubic Bone	L2,3
Iliacus	Upper 2/3 Iliac Fossa	Lesser Trochanter	Femoral L2-4

Pectinius	Pubic Ramus	Spiral Line	Femoral
Iliposoas	Joining of Psoas Major and Iliacus	Lesser Trochanter	L2-4
Piriformis	Anterior Surface of the Sacrum	Greater Trochanter	S1, S2
Obturator Internus	Inner Surface of the Obturator Membrane	Greater Trochanter	Sacral Plexus
Obturator Externus	Outer Surface of the Obturator Membrane	Greater Trochanter	Obturator
Gemellus Superior	Ischial Spine	Greater Trochanter	Sacral Plexus
Gemellus Inferior	Ischial Tuberosity	Greater Trochanter	Sacral Plexus
Quadratus Femoris	Ischial Tuberosity	Quadrate Tubercle of the Femur	Sacral Plexus
Gluteus Maximus	Outer Surface of Ilium, Sacrum and Coccyx	Iliotibial Tract, Gluteal Tubercle of the Femur	Inferior Gluteal
Gluteus Minimus	Outer Surface of the Ilium	Greater Trochanter	Superior Gluteal
Gluteus Medius	Outer Surface of the Ilium	Greater Trochanter	Superior Gluteal
Satorius	Anterior Superior Iliac Spine	Upper Medial Tibia	Femoral
Quadriceps Femoris	Anterior Inferior Iliac Spine, Femur- Lateral and Medial	Tibial Tuberosity	Femoral
Gracilis	Pubic Bone	Upper Medial Tibia	Obturator (anterior branch)
Abductor Longus	Pubic Bone	Linea Aspera	Obturator (anterior branch)
Abductor Brevis	Pubic Bone	Linea Aspera	Obturator (anterior branch)
Abductor Magnus	Pubic Bone	Entire Linea Aspera	Sciatic, Obturator
Tensor Faciae Latae	Iliac Crest	Iliotibial Band	Superior Gluteal
Biceps Femoris	Ischial Tuberosity, Linea Aspera	Head of Fibula, Lateral Condyle of Tibia	Sciatic-Tibial portion and Common Peroneal Portion
Semimembranosus	Ischial Tuberosity	Upper Medial Tibia	Sciatic-Tibial Portion
Semitendinosus	Ischial Tuberosity	Upper Medial Tibia	Sciatic-Tibial

			Portion

Musculature/Innervation Review of the Calf and Foot

Muscle	Origin	Insertion	Nerve
Tibialis Anterior	Upper 2/3 Lateral Tibia and Interosseous Membrane	1st Cuneiform and Base of 1st Metatarsal	Deep Peroneal
Extensor Digitorum Longus	Upper 2/3 Fibula and Interosseous Membrane	4 Tendons-Distal Middle Phalanges	Deep Peroneal
Extensor Hallucis Longus	Middle 1/3 of Anterior Fibula	Base of Distal Phalanx of Big Toe	Deep Peroneal
Peroneus Tertius	Distal Fibula	Base of 5th Metatarsal	Deep Peroneal
Extensor Hallucis Brevis	Dorsal Calcaneus	Extensor Digitorum Longus Tendons	Deep Peroneal
Peroneus Longus	Upper 2/3 Lateral Fibula	1st Metatarsal and 1st Cuneiform	Superficial Peroneal
Peroneus Brevis	Lateral Distal Fibula	5th Metatarsal Tuberosity	Superficial Peroneal
Soleus	Upper Shaft of Fibula	Calcaneus via Achilles Tendon	Tibial
Flexor Digitorum Longus	Middle 1/3 of Posterior Tibia	Base of Distal Phalanx of Lateral 4 Toes	Tibial
Flexor Hallucis Longus	Middle and Lower 1/3 of Posterior Tibia	Distal Phalanx of Big Toe	Tibial
Tibialis Posterior	Posterior Upper Tibia, Fibula	Navicular Bone and 1st Cuneiform	Tibial
Popliteus	Upper Posterior Tibia	Lateral Condyle of Femur	Tibial
Flexor Digitorum Brevis	Calcaneus	Middle Phalanges of Lateral 4 Toes	Medial Plantar
Abductor Hallucis	Calcaneus	Medial Proximal Phalanx of Big Toe	Medial Plantar
Abductor Digiti Brevis	Calcaneus	Lateral Proximal Phalanx of Big Toe	Lateral Plantar
Quadratus Plantae	Lateral and Medial	Tendons of Flexor	Lateral Plantar

	Side of the Calcaneus	Digitorum Longus	
Lumbricals	Tendons of Flexor Digitorum Longus	Extensor Tendons of Toes	Medial Plantar/Lateral Plantar
Flexor Hallucis Brevis	Cuboid Bone	Splits on Base of Proximal Phalanx of Big Toe	Medial Plantar
Flexor Digiti Minimi Brevis	Base of 5th Metatarsal	Base of Proximal Phalanx of Little Toe	Lateral Plantar
Abductor Hallucis	Metatarsals 2-4	Base of Proximal Phalanx of Big Toe	Lateral Plantar
Interossei	Sides of Metatarsal Bones	Base of 1st Phalanx and Extensor Tendons	Lateral Plantar

Special Report: CPR Review/Cheat Sheet

1. Risk factors of stroke:
A: heart disease
B: high red blood cell count
C: TIA's

2. Signs of a stroke:
A: alteration in consciousness
B: sudden weakness or numbness in an extremity on one side of the body
C: sudden falls
D: unexplained dizziness
E: facial paralysis
F: difficulty speaking

3. Controllable risk factors of stroke and heart attacks:
A: high blood cholesterol
B: obesity
C: TIA's
D: smoking
E: heart disease

4. Chain of survival (adults)
A: early access (911)
B: early CPR
C: early defibrillation
D: early ACLS

5. Chain of survival (pediatric)
A: prevention of injuries and arrest
B: early CPR
C: early access (911)
D: advanced care

6. Rate of compression
A: adult-about 100x per minute
B: child-about 100x per minute
C: infant-at least 100x per minute

7. Depth of compression
A: adult- 1&1/2 to 2" compression (hands overlapping)
B: child- 1 to 1&1/2" compression (only heel of one hand)
C: infant- ½ to 1" compression or 1/3 to ½ the depth of infant's chest (2 fingers)

8. Ratio of compression to ventilations

A: adult- both one and two rescuers should use a 15:2 compression to ventilation rate

B: child- both one and two rescuers should use a 5:1 compression to ventilation rate

C: infant-both one and two rescuers should use a 5:1 compression to ventilation rate

9. Rescue breath with a pulse

A: adult-5 seconds (10-12 times per minute)

B: child- 3 seconds (about 20 times per minute)

C: infant- 3 seconds (about 20 times per minute)

10. Common causes of cardiac arrest in infants and children

A: breathing emergencies

B: onset following or from illness or injury

C: heart rhythm dysfunction

Adult one-rescuer CPR

1. establish unresponsiveness, activate EMS
2. open airway-look, listen, feel
3. if breathing is inadequate or absent give 2 slow breaths
4. check carotid pulse and signs of circulation in response to the 2 rescue breaths
5. if no pulse, give cycles of 15 chest compressions
6. after 4 cycles of 15:2 check pulse
7. if no pulse cont. beginning with chest compressions

**If victim begins breathing, place in recovery position.

Child one-rescuer CPR

1. establish unresponsiveness, send second rescuer for EMS activation if available
2. open airway-look, listen, feel
3. if breathing is inadequate or absent give 2 slow breaths
4. check carotid pulse and signs of circulation in response to the 2 rescue breaths
5. if no signs of circulation are present or heart rate is less than 60 bpm with signs of poor perfusion, begin cycles of 5 chest compressions and 1 breath
6. after about 1 minute, check signs of circulation. If alone, activate EMS, then continue compression/ventilation ratio
7. if signs of circulation are present but breathing is absent or inadequate, continue rescue breathing (1 breath every 3 sec. about 20 breaths per minute)

**If victim begins breathing, place in recovery position.

Infant one-rescuer CPR

1. establish unresponsiveness, send second rescuer for EMS activation if available
2. open airway-look, listen, feel
3. if breathing is inadequate or absent give 2 slow breaths
4. check brachial pulse and signs of circulation in response to the 2 rescue breaths
5. if no signs of circulation are present or heart rate is less than 60 bpm with signs of poor perfusion, begin cycles of 5 chest compressions and 1 breath, using 2 finger technique
6. after about 1 minute, check signs of circulation. If alone, activate EMS, then continue chest compression/ventilation ratio
7. if signs of circulation are present but breathing is absent or inadequate, continue rescue breathing (1 breath every 3 sec. about 20 breaths per minute)

**If victim begins breathing, place in recovery position.

Adult-Foreign Body Airway Obstruction-Unresponsive

1. establish unresponsiveness "Are you o.k?"
2. activate EMS
3. open airway and check breathing
4. attempt to ventilate
5. give up to 5 abdominal thrusts with victim on their back
6. open airway with tongue-jaw lift followed by a finger sweep
7. repeat steps 3 through til effective, then continue CPR as necessary

Adult-Foreign Body Airway Obstruction-Responsive

1. ask "Are you choking?"
2. give abdominal thrust (chest thrusts for pregnant or obese victim)
3. repeat cycle until object is cleared or victim becomes unresponsive
4. if victim becomes unresponsive-activate EMS
5. perform tongue-jaw lift followed by finger sweep
6. open airway and try to ventilate, if still obstructed, reposition head and try again
7. give 5 abdominal thrusts with victim on their back
8. repeat steps 5-7 til breathing is effective, then continue the steps of CPR as needed

Child-Foreign Body Airway Obstruction-Unresponsive

1. establish unresponsiveness "Are you o.k?"
2. activate EMS if a second rescuer is available
3. open airway and check for breathing
4. if breathing is absent or inadequate-attempt to ventilate, if unsuccessful reposition and reattempt

5. if ventilation is unsuccessful, perform 5 abdominal thrusts with the victim on their back
6. open airway with a tongue-jaw lift, and if you see the object, remove it-no blind sweeps
7. repeat steps 3-5 until ventilation is successful, then continue the steps of CPR as needed
8. if rescuer is alone and airway obstruction is not relieved after about 1 minute, active EMS

**If victim begins breathing, place in recovery position.

Child-Foreign Body Airway Obstruction-Responsive

1. ask "Are you choking?"
2. give abdominal thrust, avoid Xyphoid
3. repeat thrusts until object is expelled or victim becomes unresponsive
4. activate EMS if a second rescuer is available
5. open airway with tongue-jaw lift, if you see the object remove it, no blind sweeps
6. open airway , attempt rescue breathing, if no chest rise, reopen airway, and try to ventilate again
7. if ventilation is unsuccessful, provide 5 abdominal thrusts with victim on their back
8. repeat steps 5-7 til effective, then provide additional CPR if necessary
9. if rescuer is alone and airway obstruction is not relieved after about 1 minute, activate EMS

**If victim begins breathing, place in recovery position.

Special Report: Pharmacology Generic/Trade Names of 50 Key Drugs in Medicine

1. Alprazolam   XANAX
2. Amitriptyline   ELAVIL
3. Amoxicillin/clavulanate potassium   AUGMENTIN
4. Betamethasone   CELESTONE
5. Bumetanide   BUMEX
6. Bupropion   WELLBUTRIN
7. Calcitriol   ROCALTROL
8. Ceforanide   PRECEF
9. Ceftazidime   FORTAZ
10. Cephalexin   KEFLEX
11. Ciprofloxacin   CIPRO
12. Clonazepam   KLONOPIN
13. Cyclobenzaprine   FLEXERIL
14. Diazepam   VALIUM
15. Dopamine   INTROPIN
16. Enalapril   VASOTEC
17. Eythromycin   E-MYCIN
18. Famotidine   PEPCID
19. Fluconazole   DiFLUCON
20. Fluoxetine   PROZAC
21. Furosemide   LASIX
22. Gentamicin   GARAMYCIN
23. Haloperidol   HALDOL
24. Hydroxyprogesterone caproate   DELALUTIN
25. Ibuprofen   MOTRIN
26. Ipratropium bromide   ATROVENT
27. Ketorolac   TORADOL
28. Lidocaine   XYLOCAINE
29. Lorazepam   ATIVAN
30. Meperidine   DEMEROL
31. Methicillin   STAPHCILLIN
32. Metoprolol   LOPRESSOR
33. Miconazole   MONISTAT
34. Nystatin   MYCOSTATIN
35. Omeprazole   PRILOSEC
36. Oxybutynin   DITROPAN
37. Oxymetholone   ANADROL
38. Pergolide   PERMAX
39. Phenytoin   DILANTIN
40. Prazepam   CENTRAX

41. Prednisone	DELTASONE
42. Procaine	NOVOCAIN
43. Promethazine	PHENERGAN
44. Propoxyphene	DARVON
45. Pseudoephedrine	SUDAFED
46. Silver sulfadiazine	SILVADENE
47. Temazepam	RESTORIL
48. Tolnaftate	TINACTIN
49. Vancomycin	VANCOCIN
50. Warfarin	COUMADIN

Special Report: What Your Test Score Will Tell You About Your IQ

Did you know that most standardized tests correlate very strongly with IQ? In fact, your general intelligence is a better predictor of your success than any other factor, and most tests intentionally measure this trait to some degree to ensure that those selected by the test are truly qualified for the test's purposes.

Before we can delve into the relation between your test score and IQ, I will first have to explain what exactly is IQ. Here's the formula:

Your IQ = 100 + (Number of standard deviations below or above the average)*15

Now, let's define standard deviations by using an example. If we have 5 people with 5 different heights, then first we calculate the average. Let's say the average was 65 inches. The standard deviation is the "average distance" away from the average of each of the members. It is a direct measure of variability - if the 5 people included Jackie Chan and Shaquille O'Neal, obviously there's a lot more variability in that group than a group of 5 sisters who are all within 6 inches in height of each other. The standard deviation uses a number to characterize the average range of difference within a group.

A convenient feature of most groups is that they have a "normal" distribution- makes sense that most things would be normal, right? Without getting into a bunch of statistical mumbo-jumbo, you just need to know that if you know the average of the group and the standard deviation, you can successfully predict someone's percentile rank in the group.

Confused? Let me give you an example. If instead of 5 people's heights, we had 100 people, we could figure out their rank in height JUST by knowing the average, standard deviation, and their height. We wouldn't need to know each person's height and manually rank them, we could just predict their rank based on three numbers.

What this means is that you can take your PERCENTILE rank that is often given with your test and relate this to your RELATIVE IQ of people taking the test - that is, your IQ relative to the people taking the test. Obviously, there's no way to know your actual IQ because the people taking a standardized test are usually not very good samples of the general population- many of those with extremely low IQ's never achieve a level of success or competency necessary to complete a typical standardized test. In fact, professional psychologists who measure IQ actually have to use non-written tests that can fairly measure the IQ of those not able to complete a traditional test.

The bottom line is to not take your test score too seriously, but it is fun to compute your "relative IQ" among the people who took the test with you. I've done the calculations below. Just look up your percentile rank in the left and then you'll see your "relative IQ" for your test in the right hand column-

Percentile Rank	Your Relative IQ		Percentile Rank	Your Relative IQ
99	135		59	103
98	131		58	103
97	128		57	103
96	126		56	102
95	125		55	102
94	123		54	102
93	122		53	101
92	121		52	101
91	120		51	100
90	119		50	100
89	118		49	100
88	118		48	99
87	117		47	99
86	116		46	98
85	116		45	98
84	115		44	98
83	114		43	97
82	114		42	97
81	113		41	97
80	113		40	96
79	112		39	96
78	112		38	95
77	111		37	95
76	111		36	95
75	110		35	94
74	110		34	94
73	109		33	93
72	109		32	93
71	108		31	93
70	108		30	92
69	107		29	92
68	107		28	91
67	107		27	91
66	106		26	90
65	106		25	90
64	105		24	89
63	105		23	89

62	105	22	88
61	104	21	88
60	104	20	87

Special Report: Retaking the Test: What Are Your Chances at Improving Your Score?

After going through the experience of taking a major test, many test takers feel that once is enough. The test usually comes during a period of transition in the test taker's life, and taking the test is only one of a series of important events. With so many distractions and conflicting recommendations, it may be difficult for a test taker to rationally determine whether or not he should retake the test after viewing his scores.

The importance of the test usually only adds to the burden of the retake decision. However, don't be swayed by emotion. There a few simple questions that you can ask yourself to guide you as you try to determine whether a retake would improve your score:

1. What went wrong? Why wasn't your score what you expected?

Can you point to a single factor or problem that you feel caused the low score? Were you sick on test day? Was there an emotional upheaval in your life that caused a distraction? Were you late for the test or not able to use the full time allotment? If you can point to any of these specific, individual problems, then a retake should definitely be considered.

2. Is there enough time to improve?

Many problems that may show up in your score report may take a lot of time for improvement. A deficiency in a particular math skill may require weeks or months of tutoring and studying to improve. If you have enough time to improve an identified weakness, then a retake should definitely be considered.

3. How will additional scores be used? Will a score average, highest score, or most recent score be used?

Different test scores may be handled completely differently. If you've taken the test multiple times, sometimes your highest score is used, sometimes your average score is computed and used, and sometimes your most recent score is used. Make sure you understand what method will be used to evaluate your scores, and use that to help you determine whether a retake should be considered.

4. Are my practice test scores significantly higher than my actual test score?

If you have taken a lot of practice tests and are consistently scoring at a much higher level than your actual test score, then you should consider a retake. However, if you've taken five practice tests and only one of your scores was higher than your actual test score, or if your practice test scores were only slightly higher than your actual test score, then it is unlikely that you will significantly increase your score.

5. Do I need perfect scores or will I be able to live with this score? Will this score still allow me to follow my dreams?

What kind of score is acceptable to you? Is your current score "good enough?" Do you have to have a certain score in order to pursue the future of your dreams? If you won't be happy with your current score, and there's no way that you could live with it, then you should consider a retake. However, don't get your hopes up. If you are looking for significant improvement, that may or may not be possible. But if you won't be happy otherwise, it is at least worth the effort.

Remember that there are other considerations. To achieve your dream, it is likely that your grades may also be taken into account. A great test score is usually not the only thing necessary to succeed. Make sure that you aren't overemphasizing the importance of a high test score.

Furthermore, a retake does not always result in a higher score. Some test takers will score lower on a retake, rather than higher. One study shows that one-fourth of test takers will achieve a significant improvement in test score, while one-sixth of test takers will actually show a decrease. While this shows that most test takers will improve, the majority will only improve their scores a little and a retake may not be worth the test taker's effort.

Finally, if a test is taken only once and is considered in the added context of good grades on the part of a test taker, the person reviewing the grades and scores may be tempted to assume that the test taker just had a bad day while taking the test, and may discount the low test score in favor of the high grades. But if the test is retaken and the scores are approximately the same, then the validity of the low scores are only confirmed. Therefore, a retake could actually hurt a test taker by definitely bracketing a test taker's score ability to a limited range.

Special Report: What is Test Anxiety and How to Overcome It?

The very nature of tests caters to some level of anxiety, nervousness or tension, just as we feel for any important event that occurs in our lives. A little bit of anxiety or nervousness can be a good thing. It helps us with motivation, and makes achievement just that much sweeter. However, too much anxiety can be a problem; especially if it hinders our ability to function and perform.

"Test anxiety," is the term that refers to the emotional reactions that some test-takers experience when faced with a test or exam. Having a fear of testing and exams is based upon a rational fear, since the test-taker's performance can shape the course of an academic career. Nevertheless, experiencing excessive fear of examinations will only interfere with the test-takers ability to perform, and his/her chances to be successful.

There are a large variety of causes that can contribute to the development and sensation of test anxiety. These include, but are not limited to lack of performance and worrying about issues surrounding the test.

Lack of Preparation

Lack of preparation can be identified by the following behaviors or situations:

Not scheduling enough time to study, and therefore cramming the night before the test or exam
Managing time poorly, to create the sensation that there is not enough time to do everything
Failing to organize the text information in advance, so that the study material consists of the entire text and not simply the pertinent information
Poor overall studying habits

Worrying, on the other hand, can be related to both the test taker, or many other factors around him/her that will be affected by the results of the test. These include worrying about:

Previous performances on similar exams, or exams in general
How friends and other students are achieving
The negative consequences that will result from a poor grade or failure

There are three primary elements to test anxiety. Physical components, which involve the same typical bodily reactions as those to acute anxiety (to be discussed below). Emotional factors have to do with fear or panic. Mental or cognitive issues concerning attention spans and memory abilities.

Physical Signals

There are many different symptoms of test anxiety, and these are not limited to mental and emotional strain. Frequently there are a range of physical signals that will let a test taker know that he/she is suffering from test anxiety. These bodily changes can include the following:

Perspiring
Sweaty palms
Wet, trembling hands
Nausea
Dry mouth
A knot in the stomach
Headache
Faintness
Muscle tension
Aching shoulders, back and neck
Rapid heart beat
Feeling too hot/cold

To recognize the sensation of test anxiety, a test-taker should monitor him/herself for the following sensations:

The physical distress symptoms as listed above
Emotional sensitivity, expressing emotional feelings such as the need to cry or laugh too much, or a sensation of anger or helplessness
A decreased ability to think, causing the test-taker to blank out or have racing thoughts that are hard to organize or control.

Though most students will feel some level of anxiety when faced with a test or exam, the majority can cope with that anxiety and maintain it at a manageable level. However, those who cannot are faced with a very real and very serious condition, which can and should be controlled for the immeasurable benefit of this sufferer.

Naturally, these sensations lead to negative results for the testing experience. The most common effects of test anxiety have to do with nervousness and mental blocking.

Nervousness

Nervousness can appear in several different levels:

The test-taker's difficulty, or even inability to read and understand the questions on the test
The difficulty or inability to organize thoughts to a coherent form
The difficulty or inability to recall key words and concepts relating to the testing questions (especially essays)
The receipt of poor grades on a test, though the test material was well known by the test taker

Conversely, a person may also experience mental blocking, which involves:

Blanking out on test questions
Only remembering the correct answers to the questions when the test has already finished.

Fortunately for test anxiety sufferers, beating these feelings, to a large degree, has to do with proper preparation. When a test taker has a feeling of preparedness, then anxiety will be dramatically lessened.

The first step to resolving anxiety issues is to distinguish which of the two types of anxiety are being suffered. If the anxiety is a direct result of a lack of preparation, this should be considered a normal reaction, and the anxiety level (as opposed to the test results) shouldn't be anything to worry about. However, if, when adequately prepared, the test-taker still panics, blanks out, or seems to overreact, this is not a fully rational reaction. While this can be considered normal too, there are many ways to combat and overcome these effects.

Remember that anxiety cannot be entirely eliminated, however, there are ways to minimize it, to make the anxiety easier to manage. Preparation is one of the best ways to minimize test anxiety. Therefore the following techniques are wise in order to best fight off any anxiety that may want to build.

To begin with, try to avoid cramming before a test, whenever it is possible. By trying to memorize an entire term's worth of information in one day, you'll be shocking your system, and not giving yourself a very good chance to absorb the information. This is an easy path to anxiety, so for those who suffer from test anxiety, cramming should not even be considered an option.

Instead of cramming, work throughout the semester to combine all of the material which is presented throughout the semester, and work on it gradually as the course goes by, making sure to master the main concepts first, leaving minor details for a week or so before the test.

To study for the upcoming exam, be sure to pose questions that may be on the examination, to gauge the ability to answer them by integrating the ideas from your texts, notes and lectures, as well as any supplementary readings.

If it is truly impossible to cover all of the information that was covered in that particular term, concentrate on the most important portions, that can be covered very well. Learn these concepts as best as possible, so that when the test comes, a goal can be made to use these concepts as presentations of your knowledge.

In addition to study habits, changes in attitude are critical to beating a struggle with test anxiety. In fact, an improvement of the perspective over the entire test-taking experience can actually help a test taker to enjoy studying and therefore improve the overall experience. Be certain not to overemphasize the significance of the grade - know that the result of the test is neither a reflection of self worth, nor is it a measure of intelligence; one grade will not predict a person's future success.

To improve an overall testing outlook, the following steps should be tried:

Keeping in mind that the most reasonable expectation for taking a test is to expect to try to demonstrate as much of what you know as you possibly can. Reminding ourselves that a test is only one test; this is not the only one, and there will be others.
The thought of thinking of oneself in an irrational, all-or-nothing term should be avoided at all costs.
A reward should be designated for after the test, so there's something to look forward to. Whether it be going to a movie, going out to eat, or simply visiting friends, schedule it in advance, and do it no matter what result is expected on the exam.

Test-takers should also keep in mind that the basics are some of the most important things, even beyond anti-anxiety techniques and studying. Never neglect the basic social, emotional and biological needs, in order to try to absorb information. In order to best achieve, these three factors must be held as just as important as the studying itself.

Study Steps

Remember the following important steps for studying:

Maintain healthy nutrition and exercise habits. Continue both your recreational activities and social pass times. These both contribute to your physical and emotional well being.

Be certain to get a good amount of sleep, especially the night before the test, because when you're overtired you are not able to perform to the best of your best ability.

Keep the studying pace to a moderate level by taking breaks when they are needed, and varying the work whenever possible, to keep the mind fresh instead of getting bored.

When enough studying has been done that all the material that can be learned has been learned, and the test taker is prepared for the test, stop studying and do something relaxing such as listening to music, watching a movie, or taking a warm bubble bath.

There are also many other techniques to minimize the uneasiness or apprehension that is experienced along with test anxiety before, during, or even after the examination. In fact, there are a great deal of things that can be done to stop anxiety from interfering with lifestyle and performance. Again, remember that anxiety will not be eliminated entirely, and it shouldn't be. Otherwise that "up" feeling for exams would not exist, and most of us depend on that sensation to perform better than usual. However, this anxiety has to be at a level that is manageable.

Of course, as we have just discussed, being prepared for the exam is half the battle right away. Attending all classes, finding out what knowledge will be expected on the exam, and knowing the exam schedules are easy steps to lowering anxiety. Keeping up with work will remove the need to cram, and efficient study habits will eliminate wasted time. Studying should be done in an ideal location for concentration, so that it is simple to become interested in the material and give it complete attention. A method such as SQ3R (Survey, Question, Read, Recite, Review) is a wonderful key to follow to make sure that the study habits are as effective as possible, especially in the case of learning from a textbook. Flashcards are great techniques for memorization. Learning to take good notes will mean that notes will be full of useful information, so that less sifting will need to be done to seek out what is pertinent for studying. Reviewing notes after class and then again on occasion will keep the information fresh in the mind. From notes that have been taken summary sheets and outlines can be made for simpler reviewing.

A study group can also be a very motivational and helpful place to study, as there will be a sharing of ideas, all of the minds can work together, to make sure that everyone understands, and the studying will be made more interesting because it will be a social occasion.

Basically, though, as long as the test-taker remains organized and self confident, with efficient study habits, less time will need to be spent studying, and higher grades will be achieved.

To become self confident, there are many useful steps. The first of these is "self talk." It has been shown through extensive research, that self-talk for students who suffer from test anxiety, should be well monitored, in order to make sure that it contributes to self confidence as opposed to sinking the student. Frequently the self talk of test-anxious students is negative or self-defeating, thinking that everyone else is smarter and faster, that they always mess up, and that if they don't do well, they'll fail the entire course. It is important to decreasing anxiety that awareness is made of self talk. Try writing any negative self thoughts and then disputing them with a positive statement instead. Begin self-encouragement as though it was a friend speaking. Repeat positive statements to help reprogram the mind to believing in successes instead of failures.

Helpful Techniques

Other extremely helpful techniques include:

Self-visualization of doing well and reaching goals
While aiming for an "A" level of understanding, don't try to "overprotect" by setting your expectations lower. This will only convince the mind to stop studying in order to meet the lower expectations.
Don't make comparisons with the results or habits of other students. These are individual factors, and different things work for different people, causing different results.
Strive to become an expert in learning what works well, and what can be done in order to improve. Consider collecting this data in a journal.
Create rewards for after studying instead of doing things before studying that will only turn into avoidance behaviors.
Make a practice of relaxing - by using methods such as progressive relaxation, self-hypnosis, guided imagery, etc - in order to make relaxation an automatic sensation.
Work on creating a state of relaxed concentration so that concentrating will take on the focus of the mind, so that none will be wasted on worrying.
Take good care of the physical self by eating well and getting enough sleep.
Plan in time for exercise and stick to this plan.

Beyond these techniques, there are other methods to be used before, during and after the test that will help the test-taker perform well in addition to overcoming anxiety.

Before the exam comes the academic preparation. This involves establishing a study schedule and beginning at least one week before the actual date of the test. By doing this, the anxiety of not having enough time to study for the test will be automatically eliminated. Moreover, this will make the studying a much more effective experience, ensuring that the learning will be an easier process. This relieves much undue pressure on the test-taker.

Summary sheets, note cards, and flash cards with the main concepts and examples of these main concepts should be prepared in advance of the actual studying time. A topic should never be eliminated from this process. By omitting a topic because it isn't expected to be on the test is only setting up the test-taker for anxiety should it actually appear on the exam. Utilize the course syllabus for laying out the topics that should be studied. Carefully go over the notes that were made in class, paying special attention to any of the issues that the professor took special care to emphasize while lecturing in class. In the textbooks, use the chapter review, or if possible, the chapter tests, to begin your review.

It may even be possible to ask the instructor what information will be covered on the exam, or what the format of the exam will be (for example, multiple choice, essay, free form, true-false). Additionally, see if it is possible to find out how many questions will be on the test. If a review sheet or sample test has been offered by the professor, make good use of it, above anything else, for the preparation for the test. Another great resource for getting to know the examination is reviewing tests from previous semesters. Use these tests to review, and aim to achieve a 100% score on each of the possible topics. With a few exceptions, the goal that you set for yourself is the highest one that you will reach.

Take all of the questions that were assigned as homework, and rework them to any other possible course material. The more problems reworked, the more skill and confidence will form as a result. When forming the solution to a problem, write out each of the steps. Don't simply do head work. By doing as many steps on paper as possible, much clarification and therefore confidence will be formed. Do this with as many homework problems as possible, before checking the answers. By checking the answer after each problem, a reinforcement will exist, that will not be on the exam. Study situations should be as exam-like as possible, to prime the test-taker's system for the experience. By waiting to check the answers at the end, a psychological advantage will be formed, to decrease the stress factor.

Another fantastic reason for not cramming is the avoidance of confusion in concepts, especially when it comes to mathematics. 8-10 hours of study will become one hundred percent more effective if it is spread out over a week or at least several days, instead of doing it all in one sitting. Recognize that the human brain requires time in order to assimilate new material, so frequent breaks and a span of study time over several days will be much more beneficial.

Additionally, don't study right up until the point of the exam. Studying should stop a minimum of one hour before the exam begins. This allows the brain to rest and put things in their proper order. This will also provide the time to become as relaxed as possible when going into the examination room. The test-taker will also have time to eat well and eat sensibly. Know that the brain needs food as much as the rest of the body. With enough food and enough sleep, as well as a relaxed attitude, the body and the mind are primed for success.

Avoid any anxious classmates who are talking about the exam. These students only spread anxiety, and are not worth sharing the anxious sentimentalities.

Before the test also involves creating a positive attitude, so mental preparation should also be a point of concentration. There are many keys to creating a positive attitude. Should fears become rushing in, make a visualization of taking the exam, doing well, and seeing an A written on the paper. Write out a list of affirmations that will bring a feeling of confidence, such as "I am doing well in my English class," "I studied well and know my material," "I enjoy this class." Even if the affirmations aren't believed at first, it sends a positive message to the subconscious which will result in an alteration of the overall belief system, which is the system that creates reality.

If a sensation of panic begins, work with the fear and imagine the very worst! Work through the entire scenario of not passing the test, failing the entire course, and dropping out of school, followed by not getting a job, and pushing a shopping cart through the dark alley where you'll live. This will place things into perspective! Then, practice deep breathing and create a visualization of the opposite situation - achieving an "A" on the exam, passing the entire course, receiving the degree at a graduation ceremony.

On the day of the test, there are many things to be done to ensure the best results, as well as the most calm outlook. The following stages are suggested in order to maximize test-taking potential:

Begin the examination day with a moderate breakfast, and avoid any coffee or beverages with caffeine if the test taker is prone to jitters. Even people who are used to managing caffeine can feel jittery or light-headed when it is taken on a test day.
Attempt to do something that is relaxing before the examination begins. As last minute cramming clouds the mastering of overall concepts, it is better to use this time to create a calming outlook.

Be certain to arrive at the test location well in advance, in order to provide time to select a location that is away from doors, windows and other distractions, as well as giving enough time to relax before the test begins.

Keep away from anxiety generating classmates who will upset the sensation of stability and relaxation that is being attempted before the exam.

Should the waiting period before the exam begins cause anxiety, create a self-distraction by reading a light magazine or something else that is relaxing and simple.

During the exam itself, read the entire exam from beginning to end, and find out how much time should be allotted to each individual problem. Once writing the exam, should more time be taken for a problem, it should be abandoned, in order to begin another problem. If there is time at the end, the unfinished problem can always be returned to and completed.

Read the instructions very carefully - twice - so that unpleasant surprises won't follow during or after the exam has ended.

When writing the exam, pretend that the situation is actually simply the completion of homework within a library, or at home. This will assist in forming a relaxed atmosphere, and will allow the brain extra focus for the complex thinking function.

Begin the exam with all of the questions with which the most confidence is felt. This will build the confidence level regarding the entire exam and will begin a quality momentum. This will also create encouragement for trying the problems where uncertainty resides.

Going with the "gut instinct" is always the way to go when solving a problem. Second guessing should be avoided at all costs. Have confidence in the ability to do well.

For essay questions, create an outline in advance that will keep the mind organized and make certain that all of the points are remembered. For multiple choice, read every answer, even if the correct one has been spotted - a better one may exist.

Continue at a pace that is reasonable and not rushed, in order to be able to work carefully. Provide enough time to go over the answers at the end, to check for small errors that can be corrected.

Should a feeling of panic begin, breathe deeply, and think of the feeling of the body releasing sand through its pores. Visualize a calm, peaceful place, and include all of the sights, sounds and sensations of this image. Continue the deep breathing, and take a few minutes to continue this with closed eyes. When all is well again, return to the test.

If a "blanking" occurs for a certain question, skip it and move on to the next question. There will be time to return to the other question later. Get everything done that can be done, first, to guarantee all the grades that can be compiled, and to build all of the confidence possible. Then return to the weaker questions to build the marks from there.

Remember, one's own reality can be created, so as long as the belief is there, success will follow. And remember: anxiety can happen later, right now, there's an exam to be written!

After the examination is complete, whether there is a feeling for a good grade or a bad grade, don't dwell on the exam, and be certain to follow through on the reward that was promised...and enjoy it! Don't dwell on any mistakes that have been made, as there is nothing that can be done at this point anyway.

Additionally, don't begin to study for the next test right away. Do something relaxing for a while, and let the mind relax and prepare itself to begin absorbing information again.

From the results of the exam - both the grade and the entire experience, be certain to learn from what has gone on. Perfect studying habits and work some more on confidence in order to make the next examination experience even better than the last one.

Learn to avoid places where openings occurred for laziness, procrastination and day dreaming.

Use the time between this exam and the next one to better learn to relax, even learning to relax on cue, so that any anxiety can be controlled during the next exam. Learn how to relax the body. Slouch in your chair if that helps. Tighten and then relax all of the different muscle groups, one group at a time, beginning with the feet and then working all the way up to the neck and face. This will ultimately relax the muscles more than they were to begin with. Learn how to breathe deeply and comfortably, and focus on this breathing going in and out as a relaxing thought. With every exhale, repeat the word "relax."

As common as test anxiety is, it is very possible to overcome it. Make yourself one of the test-takers who overcome this frustrating hindrance.

Special Report: How to Overcome Your Fear of Math

If this article started by saying "Math," many of us would feel a shiver crawl up our spines, just by reading that simple word. Images of torturous years in those crippling desks of the math classes can become so vivid to our consciousness that we can almost smell those musty textbooks, and see the smudges of the #2 pencils on our fingers.

If you are still a student, feeling the impact of these sometimes overwhelming classroom sensations, you are not alone if you get anxious at just the thought of taking that compulsory math course. Does your heart beat just that much faster when you have to split the bill for lunch among your friends with a group of your friends? Do you truly believe that you simply don't have the brain for math? Certainly you're good at other things, but math just simply isn't one of them? Have you ever avoided activities, or other school courses because they appear to involve mathematics, with which you're simply not comfortable?

If any one or more of these "symptoms" can be applied to you, you could very well be suffering from a very real condition called "Math Anxiety."

It's not at all uncommon for people to think that they have some sort of math disability or allergy, when in actuality, their block is a direct result of the way in which they were taught math!

In the late 1950's with the dawning of the space age, New Math - a new "fuzzy math" reform that focuses on higher-order thinking, conceptual understanding and solving problems - took the country by storm. It's now becoming ever more clear that teachers were not supplied with the correct, practical and effective way in which they should be teaching new math so that students will understand the methods comfortably. So is it any wonder that so many students struggled so deeply, when their teachers were required to change their entire math systems without the foundation of proper training? Even if you have not been personally, directly affected by that precise event, its impact is still as rampant as ever.

Basically, the math teachers of today are either the teachers who began teaching the new math in the first place (without proper training) or they are the students of the math teachers who taught new math without proper training. Therefore, unless they had a unique, exceptional teacher, their primary, consistent examples of teaching math have been teachers using methods that are not conducive to the general understanding of the entire class. This explains why your discomfort (or fear) of math is not at all rare.

It is very clear why being called up to the chalk board to solve a math problem is such a common example of a terrifying situation for students - and it has very little to do with a fear of being in front of the class. Most of us have had a minimum of one humiliating experience while standing with chalk dusted fingers, with the eyes of every math student piercing through us. These are the images that haunt us all the way through adulthood. But it does not mean that we cannot learn math. It just means that we could be developing a solid case of math anxiety.

But what exactly is math anxiety? It's an very strong emotional sensation of anxiety, panic, or fear that people feel when they think about or must apply their ability to understand mathematics. Sufferers of math anxiety frequently believe that they are incapable of doing activities or taking classes that involve math skills. In fact, some people with math anxiety have developed such a fear that it has become a phobia; aptly named math phobia.

The incidence of math anxiety, especially among college students, but also among high school students, has risen considerably over the last 10 years, and currently this increase shows no signs of slowing down. Frequently students will even chose their college majors and programs based specifically on how little math will be compulsory for the completion of the degree.

The prevalence of math anxiety has become so dramatic on college campuses that many of these schools have special counseling programs that are designed to assist math anxious students to deal with their discomfort and their math problems.

Math anxiety itself is not an intellectual problem, as many people have been lead to believe; it is, in fact, an emotional problem that stems from improper math teaching techniques that have slowly built and reinforced these feelings. However, math anxiety can result in an intellectual problem when its symptoms interfere with a person's ability to learn and understand math.

The fear of math can cause a sort of "glitch" in the brain that can cause an otherwise clever person to stumble over even the simplest of math problems. A study by Dr. Mark H. Ashcraft of Cleveland State University in Ohio showed that college students who usually perform well, but who suffer from math anxiety, will suffer from fleeting lapses in their working memory when they are asked to perform even the most basic mental arithmetic. These same issues regarding memory were not present in the same students when they were required to answer questions that did not involve numbers. This very clearly demonstrated that the memory phenomenon is quite specific to only math.

So what exactly is it that causes this inhibiting math anxiety? Unfortunately it is not as simple as one answer, since math anxiety doesn't have one specific cause. Frequently math anxiety can result of a student's either negative experience or embarrassment with math or a math teacher in previous years.

These circumstances can prompt the student to believe that he or she is somehow deficient in his or her math abilities. This belief will consistently lead to a poor performance in math tests and courses in general, leading only to confirm the beliefs of the student's inability. This particular phenomenon is referred to as the "self-fulfilling prophecy" by the psychological community. Math anxiety will result in poor performance, rather than it being the other way around.

Dr. Ashcraft stated that math anxiety is a "It's a learned, almost phobic, reaction to math," and that it is not only people prone to anxiety, fear, or panic who can develop math anxiety. The image alone of doing math problems can send the blood pressure and heart rate to race, even in the calmest person.

The study by Dr. Ashcraft and his colleague Elizabeth P. Kirk, discovered that students who suffered from math anxiety were frequently stumped by issues of even the most basic math rules, such as "carrying over" a number, when performing a sum, or "borrowing" from a number when doing a subtraction. Lapses such as this occurred only on working memory questions involving numbers.

To explain the problem with memory, Ashcraft states that when math anxiety begins to take its effect, the sufferer experiences a rush of thoughts, leaving little room for the focus required to perform even the simplest of math problems. He stated that "you're draining away the energy you need for solving the problem by worrying about it."

The outcome is a "vicious cycle," for students who are sufferers of math anxiety. As math anxiety is developed, the fear it promotes stands in the way of learning, leading to a decrease in self-confidence in the ability to perform even simple arithmetic.

A large portion of the problem lies in the ways in which math is taught to students today. In the US, students are frequently taught the rules of math, but rarely will they learn why a specific approach to a math problems work. Should students be provided with a foundation of "deeper understanding" of math, it may prevent the development of phobias.

Another study that was published in the Journal of Experimental Psychology by Dr. Jamie Campbell and Dr. Qilin Xue of the University of Saskatchewan in Saskatoon, Canada, reflected the same concepts. The researchers in this study looked at university students who were educated in Canada and China, discovering that the Chinese students could generally outperform the Canadian-educated students when it came to solving complex math problems involving procedural knowledge - the ability to know how to solve a math problem, instead of simply having ideas memorized.

A portion of this result seemed to be due to the use of calculators within both elementary and secondary schools; while Canadians frequently used them, the Chinese students did not.

However, calculators were not the only issue. Since Chinese-educated students also outperformed Canadian-educated students in complex math, it is suggested that cultural factors may also have an impact. However, the short-cut of using the calculator may hinder the development of the problem solving skills that are key to performing well in math.

Though it is critical that students develop such fine math skills, it is easier said than done. It would involve an overhaul of the training among all elementary and secondary educators, changing the education major in every college.

Math Myths

One problem that contributes to the progression of math anxiety, is the belief of many math myths. These erroneous math beliefs include the following:

Men are better in math than women - however, research has failed to demonstrate that there is any difference in math ability between the sexes. There is a single best way to solve a math problem - however, the majority of math problems can be solved in a number of different ways. By saying that there is only one way to solve a math problem, the thinking and creative skills of the student are held back.

Some people have a math mind, and others do not - in truth, the majority of people have much more potential for their math capabilities than they believe of themselves.

It is a bad thing to count by using your fingers - counting by using fingers has actually shown that an understanding of arithmetic has been established. People who are skilled in math can do problems quickly in their heads - in actuality, even math professors will review their example problems before they teach them in their classes.

The anxieties formed by these myths can frequently be perpetuated by a range of mind games that students seem to play with themselves. These math mind games include the following beliefs:

I don't perform math fast enough - actually everyone has a different rate at which he or she can learn. The speed of the solving of math problems is not important as long as the student can solve it.

I don't have the mind for math - this belief can inhibit a student's belief in him or herself, and will therefore interfere with the student's real ability to learn math.

I got the correct answer, but it was done the wrong way - there is no single best way to complete a math problem. By believing this, a student's creativity and overall understanding of math is hindered.

If I can get the correct answer, then it is too simple - students who suffer from math anxiety frequently belittle their own abilities when it comes to their math capabilities.

Math is unrelated to my "real" life - by freeing themselves of the fear of math, math anxiety sufferers are only limiting their choices and freedoms for the rest of their life.

Fortunately, there are many ways to help those who suffer from math anxiety. Since math anxiety is a learned, psychological response to doing or thinking about math, that interferes with the sufferer's ability to understand and perform math, it is not at all a reflection of the sufferer's true math sills and abilities.

Helpful Strategies

Many strategies and therapies have been developed to help students to overcome their math anxious responses. Some of these helpful strategies include the following:

Reviewing and learning basic arithmetic principles, techniques and methods. Frequently math anxiety is a result of the experience of many students with early negative situations, and these students have never truly developed a strong base in basic arithmetic, especially in the case of multiplication and fractions. Since math is a discipline that is built on an accumulative foundation, where the concepts are built upon gradually from simpler concepts, a student who has not achieved a solid basis in arithmetic will experience difficulty in learning higher order math. Taking a remedial math course, or a short math course that focuses on arithmetic can often make a considerable difference in reducing the anxious response that math anxiety sufferers have with math.

Becoming aware of any thoughts, actions and feelings that are related to math and responses to math. Math anxiety has a different effect on different students. Therefore it is very important to become familiar with any reactions that the math anxiety sufferer may have about him/herself and the situation when math has been encountered. If the sufferer becomes aware of any irrational or unrealistic thoughts, it's possible to better concentrate on replacing these thoughts with more positive and realistic ones.

Find help! Math anxiety, as we've mentioned, is a learned response, that is reinforced repeatedly over a period of time, and is therefore not something that can be eliminated instantaneously. Students can more effectively reduce their anxious responses with the help of many different services that are readily available. Seeking the assistance of a psychologist or counselor, especially one with a specialty in math anxiety, can assist the sufferer in performing an analysis of his/her psychological response to math, as well as learning anxiety management skills, and developing effective coping strategies. Other great tools are tutors, classes that teach better abilities to take better notes in math class, and other math learning aids.

Learning the mathematic vocabulary will instantly provide a better chance for understanding new concepts. One major issue among students is the lack of understanding of the terms and vocabulary that are common jargon within math classes. Typically math classes will utilize words in a completely different way from the way in which they are utilized in all other subjects. Students easily mistake their lack of understanding the math terms with their mathematical abilities.

Learning anxiety reducing techniques and methods for anxiety management. Anxiety greatly interferes with a student's ability to concentrate, think clearly, pay attention, and remember new concepts. When these same students can learn to relax, using anxiety management techniques, the student can regain his or her ability to control his or her emotional and physical symptoms of anxiety that interfere with the capabilities of mental processing.

Working on creating a positive overall attitude about mathematics. Looking at math with a positive attitude will reduce anxiety through the building of a positive attitude.

Learning to self-talk in a positive way. Pep talking oneself through a positive self talk can greatly assist in overcoming beliefs in math myths or the mind games that may be played. Positive self-talking is an effective way to replace the negative thoughts - the ones that create the anxiety. Even if the sufferer doesn't believe the statements at first, it plants a positive seed in the subconscious, and allows a positive outlook to grow.

Beyond this, students should learn effective math class, note taking and studying techniques. Typically, the math anxious students will avoid asking questions to save themselves from embarrassment. They will sit in the back of classrooms, and refrain from seeking assistance from the professor. Moreover, they will put off studying for math until the very last moment, since it causes them such substantial discomfort. Alone, or a combination of these negative behaviors work only to reduce the anxiety of the students, but in reality, they are actually building a substantially more intense anxiety.

There are many different positive behaviors that can be adopted by math anxious students, so that they can learn to better perform within their math classes.

Sit near the front of the class. This way, there will be fewer distractions, and there will be more of a sensation of being a part of the topic of discussion. If any questions arise, ASK! If one student has a question, then there are certain to be others who have the same question but are too nervous to ask - perhaps because they have not yet learned how to deal with their own math anxiety.

Seek extra help from the professor after class or during office hours.

Prepare, prepare, prepare - read textbook material before the class, do the homework and work out any problems available within the textbook. Math skills are developed through practice and repetition, so the more practice and repetition, the better the math skills.

Review the material once again after class, to repeat it another time, and to reinforce the new concepts that were learned.

Beyond these tactics that can be taken by the students themselves, teachers and parents need to know that they can also have a large impact on the reduction of math anxiety within students.

As parents and teachers, there is a natural desire to help students to learn and understand how they will one day utilize different math techniques within their everyday lives. But when the student or teacher displays the symptoms of a person who has had nightmarish memories regarding math, where hesitations then develop in the instruction of students, these fears are automatically picked up by the students and commonly adopted as their own.

However, it is possible for teachers and parents to move beyond their own fears to better educate students by overcoming their own hesitations and learning to enjoy math.

Begin by adopting the outlook that math is a beautiful, imaginative or living thing. Of course, we normally think of mathematics as numbers that can be added or subtracted, multiplied or divided, but that is simply the beginning of it.

By thinking of math as something fun and imaginative, parents and teachers can teach children different ways to manipulate numbers, for example in balancing a checkbook. Parents rarely tell their children that math is everywhere around us; in nature, art, and even architecture. Usually, this is because they were never shown these relatively simple connections. But that pattern can break very simply through the participation of parents and teachers.

The beauty and hidden wonders of mathematics can easily be emphasized through a focus that can open the eyes of students to the incredible mathematical patterns that arise everywhere within the natural world. Observations and discussions can be made into things as fascinating as spider webs, leaf patterns, sunflowers and even coastlines. This makes math not only beautiful, but also inspiring and (dare we say) fun!

Pappas Method

For parents and teachers to assist their students in discovering the true wonders of mathematics, the techniques of Theoni Pappas can easily be applied, as per her popular and celebrated book "Fractals, Googols and Other Mathematical Tales." Pappas used to be a math phobia sufferer and created a fascinating step-by-step program for parents and teachers to use in order to teach students the joy of math.

Her simple, constructive step-by-step program goes as follows:

Don't let your fear of math come across to your kids - Parents must be careful not to perpetuate the mathematical myth - that math is only for specially talented "math types." Strive not to make comments like; "they don't like math" or "I have never been good at math." When children overhear comments like these from their primary role models they begin to dread math before even considering a chance of experiencing its wonders. It is important to encourage your children to read and explore the rich world of mathematics, and to practice mathematics without imparting negative biases.

Don't immediately associate math with computation (counting) - It is very important to realize that math is not just numbers and computations, but a realm of exciting ideas that touch every part of our lives -from making a telephone call to how the hair grows on someone's head. Take your children outside and point out real objects that display math concepts. For example, show them the symmetry of a leaf or angles on a building. Take a close look at the spirals in a spider web or intricate patterns of a snowflake.

Help your child understand why math is important - Math improves problem solving, increases competency and should be applied in different ways. It's the same as reading. You can learn the basics of reading without ever enjoying a novel. But, where's the excitement in that? With math, you could stop with the basics. But why when there is so much more to be gained by a fuller Understanding? Life is so much more enriching when we go beyond the basics. Stretch your children's minds to become involved in mathematics in ways that will not only be practical but also enhance their lives.

Make math as "hands on" as possible - Mathematicians participate in mathematics. To really experience math encourage your child to dig in and tackle problems in creative ways. Help them learn how to manipulate numbers using concrete references they understand as well as things they can see or touch. Look for patterns everywhere, explore shapes and symmetries. How many octagons do you see each day on the way to the grocery store? Play math puzzles and games and then encourage your child to try to invent their own. And, whenever possible, help your child realize a mathematical conclusion with real and tangible results. For example, measure out a full glass of juice with a measuring cup and then ask your child to drink half. Measure what is left. Does it measure half of a cup?

Read books that make math exciting:

Fractals, Googols and Other Mathematical Tales introduces an animated cat who explains fractals, tangrams and other mathematical concepts you've probably never heard of to children in terms they can understand. This book can double as a great text book by using one story per lesson.

A Wrinkle in Time is a well-loved classic, combining fantasy and science.

The Joy of Mathematics helps adults explore the beauty of mathematics that is all around.

The Math Curse is an amusing book for 4-8 year olds.

The Gnarly Gnews is a free, humorous bi-monthly newsletter on mathematics.

The Phantom Tollbooth is an Alice in Wonderland-style adventure into the worlds of words and numbers.

Use the internet to help your child explore the fascinating world of mathematics.

Web Math provides a powerful set of math-solvers that gives you instant answers to the stickiest problems.

Math League has challenging math materials and contests for fourth grade and above.

Silver Burdett Ginn Mathematics offers Internet-based math activities for grades K-6.

The Gallery of Interactive Geometry is full of fascinating, interactive geometry activities.

Math is very much like a language of its own. And like any second language, it will get rusty if it is not practiced enough. For that reason, students should always be looking into new ways to keep understanding and brushing up on their math skills, to be certain that foundations do not crumble, inhibiting the learning of new levels of math.

There are many different books, services and websites that have been developed to take the fear out of math, and to help even the most uncertain student develop self confidence in his or her math capabilities.

There is no reason for math or math classes to be a frightening experience, nor should it drive a student crazy, making them believe that they simply don't have the "math brain" that is needed to solve certain problems.

There are friendly ways to tackle such problems and it's all a matter of dispelling myths and creating a solid math foundation.

Concentrate on re-learning the basics and feeling better about yourself in math, and you'll find that the math brain you've always wanted, was there all along.

Special Report: Difficult Patients

Every professional will eventually get a difficult patient on their list of responsibilities. These patients can be mentally, physically, and emotionally combative in many different environments. Consequently, care of these patients should be conducted in a manner for personal and self-protection of the professional. Some of the key guidelines are as follows:

1. Never allow yourself to be cornered in a room with the patient positioned between you and the door.
2. Don't escalate the tension with verbal bantering. Basically, don't argue with the patient or resident.
3. Ask permission before performing any normal tasks in a patient's room whenever possible.
4. Discuss your concerns with nursing staff. Consult the floor supervisor if necessary, especially when safety is an issue.
5. Get help from other support staff when offering care. Get a witness if you are anticipating abuse of any kind.
6. Remove yourself from the situation if you are concerned about your personal safety at all times.
7. If attacked, defend yourself with the force necessary for self-protection and attempt to separate from the patient.
8. Be aware of the patient's medical and mental history prior to entering the patient's room.
9. Don't put yourself in a position to be hurt.
10. Get the necessary help for all transfers, bathing and dressing activities from other staff members for difficult patients.
11. Respect the resident and patient's personal property.
12. Get assistance quickly, via the call bell or vocal projection, if a situation becomes violent or abuse.
13. Immediately seek medical treatment if injured.
14. Fill out an incident report for proper documentation of the occurrence.
15. Protect other patients from abusive behavior.

Special Report: Guidelines for Standard Precautions

Standard precautions are precautions taken to avoid contracting various diseases and preventing the spread of disease to those who have compromised immunity. Some of these diseases include human immunodeficiency virus (HIV), acquired immunodeficiency syndrome (AIDS), and hepatitis B (HBV). Standard precautions are needed since many diseases do not display signs or symptoms in their early stages. Standard precautions mean to treat all body fluids/ substances as if they were contaminated. These body fluids include but are not limited to the following blood, semen, vaginal secretions, breast milk, amniotic fluid, feces, urine, peritoneal fluid, synovial fluid, cerebrospinal fluid, secretions from the nasal and oral cavities, and lacrimal and sweat gland excretions. This means that standard precautions should be used with all patients.

1. A shield for the eyes and face must be used if there is a possibility of splashes from blood and body fluids.
2. If possibility of blood or body fluids being splashed on clothing, you must wear a plastic apron.
3. Gloves must be worn if you could possibly come in contact with blood or body fluids. They are also needed if you are going to touch something that may have come in contact with blood or body fluids.
4. Hands must be washed even if you were wearing gloves. Hands must be washed and gloves must be changed between patients. Wash hands with at a dime size amount of soap and warm water for about 30 seconds. Singing "Mary had a little lamb" is approximately 30 seconds.
5. Blood and body fluid spills must be cleansed and disinfected using a solution of one part bleach to 10 parts water or your hospitals accepted method.
6. Used needles must be separated from clean needles. Throw both the needle and the syringe away in the sharps' container. The sharps' container is mad of puncture proof material.
7. Take extra care in performing high-risk activities that include puncturing the skin and cutting the skin.
8. CPR equipment to be used in a hospital must include resuscitation bags and mouthpieces.

Special precautions must be taken to dispose of biomedical waste. Biomedical waste includes but is not limited to the following laboratory waste, pathology waste, liquid waste from suction, all sharp object, bladder catheters, chest tubes, IV tubes, and drainage containers. Biomedical waste is removed from a facility by trained biomedical waste disposers.

The health care professional is legally and ethically responsible for adhering to standard precautions. They may prevent you from contracting a fatal disease or from a patient contracting a disease from you that could be deadly.

Special Report: Basic Review of Types of Fractures

A fracture is defined as a break in a bone that may sometimes involve cartilaginous structures. A fracture can be classified according to its cause or the type of break. The following definitions are used to describe breaks.

1. Traumatic fracture – break in a bone resulting from injury
2. Spontaneous fracture – break in a bone resulting from disease
3. Pathologic fracture – another name for a spontaneous fracture
4. Compound fracture – occurs when fracture bone is exposed to the outside by an opening in the skin
5. Simple fracture - occurs when a break is contained within the skin
6. Greenstick fracture - a traumatic break that is incomplete and occurs on the convex surface of the bend in the bone
7. Fissured fracture – a traumatic break that involves an incomplete longitudinal break
8. Comminuted fracture – a traumatic break that involves a complete fracture that results in several bony fragments
9. Transverse fracture – a traumatic break that is complete and occurs at a right angle to the axis of the bone
10. Oblique fracture- a traumatic break that occurs at an angle other than a right angel to the axis of the bone.
11. Spiral fracture – a traumatic break that occurs by twisting a bone with extreme force

A compound fracture is much more dangerous than a simple break. This is due to the break in skin that can allow microorganisms to infect the injured tissue. When a fracture occurs, blood vessels within the bone and its periosteum are disrupted. The periosteum, covering of fibrous connective tissue on the surface of the bone, may also be damaged or torn.

Special Report: Additional Bonus Material

Due to our efforts to try to keep this book to a manageable length, we've created a link that will give you access to all of your additional bonus material.

Please visit http://www.mo-media.com/psb/bonussesho to access the information.